THE
CLEAN
PLATE

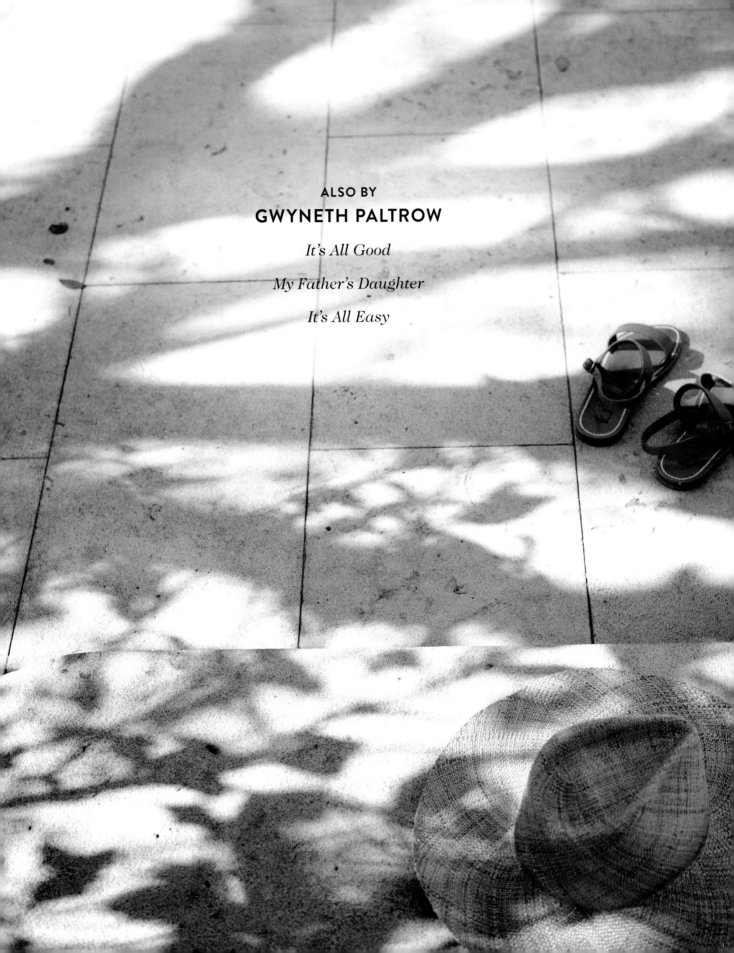

ALSO BY
GWYNETH PALTROW

It's All Good

My Father's Daughter

It's All Easy

THE

Eat, Reset, Heal

CLEAN

GWYNETH PALTROW

PLATE

PHOTOGRAPHS BY DITTE ISAGER

goop
press

GRAND CENTRAL
Life & Style
NEW YORK • BOSTON

Grand Central Life & Style
Hachette Book Group
1290 Avenue of the Americas, New York, NY 10104
grandcentrallifeandstyle.com
twitter.com/grandcentralpub

First Edition: January 2019

Grand Central Life & Style is an imprint of Grand Central Publishing. The Grand Central Life & Style name and logo are trademarks of Hachette Book Group, Inc.

The publisher is not responsible for websites (or their content) that are not owned by the publisher.

The Hachette Speakers Bureau provides a wide range of authors for speaking events. To find out more, go to www.hachettespeakersbureau.com or call (866) 376-6591.

Library of Congress Control Number: 2018953666

ISBNs: 978-1-5387-3046-1 (hardcover),
978-1-5387-3047-8 (ebook)

Printed in the United States of America

Worzalla

10 9 8 7 6 5 4 3 2

For Brad,
my favorite dinner companion,
who taught me that
it is never too late
to make a clean start.

And for Apple, Moses, Isabella,
and Brody.

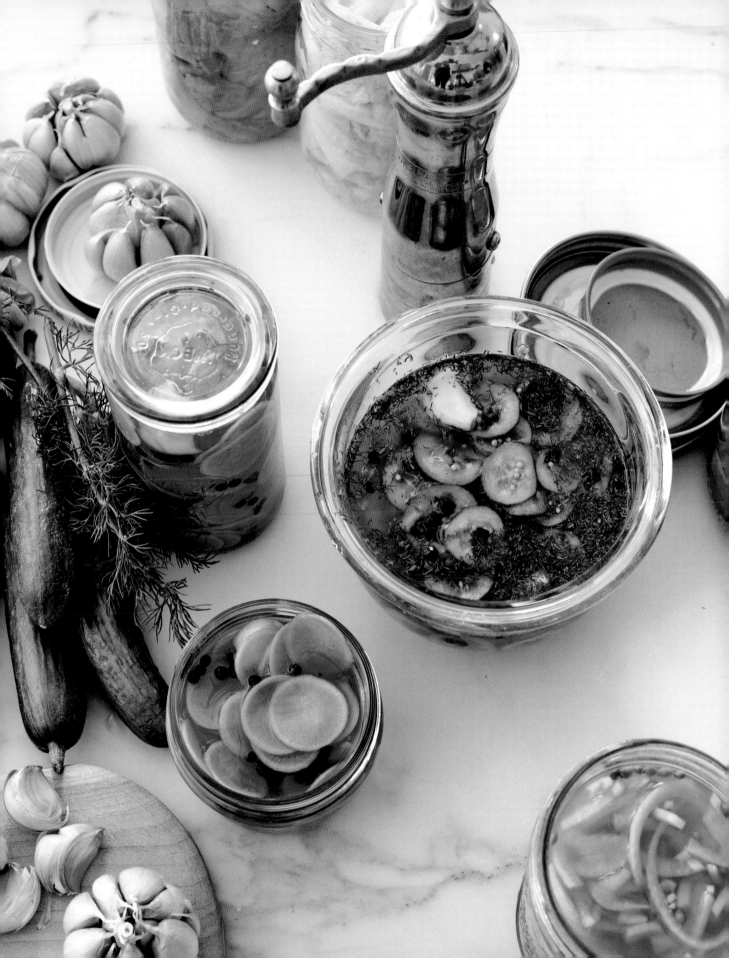

CONTENTS

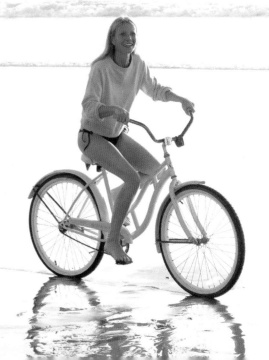

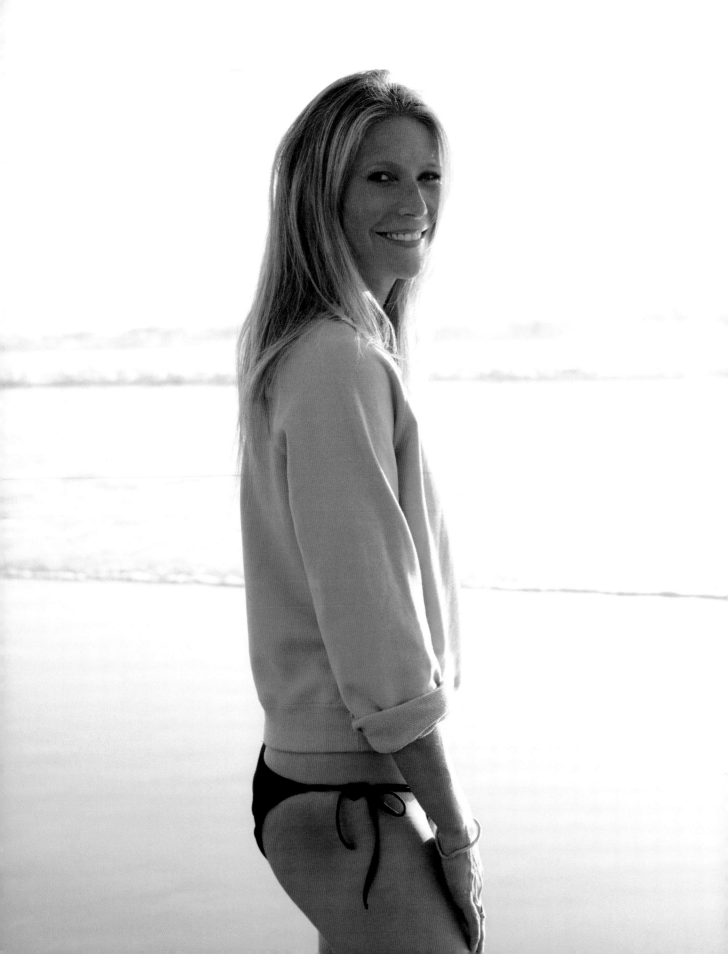

INTRODUCTION

Life is messy. It's supposed to be. Everyone I know, myself included, is juggling too many things. But we also don't want to be told to slow down or to give something up. If anything, I hear from friends, already with full plates, about other projects they're looking to take on: the next school event they've signed on to work, boards they've recently joined, causes they want to champion, or new relationships they're investing time in. In the background of all this productivity and duty and excitement, I hear a common refrain that's all too relatable. It's typically pushed to the side, downplayed, or simply drowned out: *I don't feel...great.*

There's so much that's outside our control, but how do we begin to claim some autonomy over our own health and well-being? What levers can we pull that can make a difference in how we feel? And how do we do this without sacrificing, without saying "no" to the things we want to say "yes" to, without pulling back at the office or at home or anywhere else?

Everyone's toolbox for optimal wellness looks different. For me, the most powerful reset button is food. I don't know any magic bullets, but eating clean comes close. (Although I have to say that good sleep is high up on the list for me, too.) There's a marked difference, for the better, in how I feel, and to a lesser degree how I look, when I'm eating at least fairly clean.

When I say "clean," a lot of people picture me living off foods like kale, oat milk, kelp powder, wheatgrass—and who knows what other foods that I would never actually eat. I also typically do a cleanse only once a year, which is not about punishing my body for enjoying things like burgers and whiskey the rest of the year. Eating clean as a baseline, or full-on, for a set period of time isn't a moral choice, and it shouldn't have to feel like an act of deprivation.

Of course, I see why it looks that way. At the core of almost every cleanse I've tried that's worked—in at least giving me more energy—is cutting out a specified set of ingredients from your diet for a set amount of time. The ingredients excluded on most cleanses are processed foods and sugars, gluten, dairy, red meat, soy, peanuts, nightshades, alcohol, and caffeine. In general, these foods are more likely to be associated with sensitivities, inflammatory reactions, and

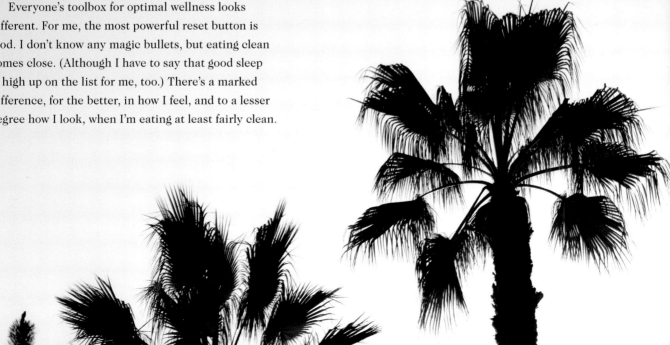

digestive issues. My good friend Dr. Alejandro Junger (more from him on page 231) has called them "toxic triggers," which, he explains, can compromise the integrity of the gut lining and health of the intestinal flora. You may have heard the functional medicine phrase "leaky gut"—a condition in which the gut lining is perforated—which is thought to be connected to a host of health issues. Dr. Junger has explained to me that the gut is the most complex system in the body—it processes food, absorbs nutrients, eliminates toxins, helps to regulate mood, and is home to about 70 percent of our immune system and a nervous system larger than the one inside our skulls.

It makes sense: When the gut is off, the body isn't running optimally. And when people eliminate or at least limit their toxic triggers, the results can be dramatic and all-encompassing—some notice improvements in their skin complexion, others less bloat, and some a more level mood, for starters. But maybe the most rewarding effect of switching to a cleaner diet is the ability to better tune into what your body likes and what it prefers to do without. If you don't know if you're sensitive to cheese or nightshades like eggplants, removing basic inflammatory triggers for an extended period of time (twenty-one days seems to be a threshold) gives you a cleaner slate to find out. After, assuming you have the time and patience to reintroduce food groups one at a time, you can see how each ingredient affects you or not. (I also recommend getting tested for food sensitivities and allergies if it's a concern.)

Admittedly, part of the reason eating clean is associated with deprivation is that, once you remove things like mozzarella and pasta, the food offerings on the table have not traditionally been all that exciting. This was partly the impetus behind my cookbook *It's All Good*—to find a way to make mealtimes fun and full of taste and flavor, without falling back on the classic comfort foods.

For *The Clean Plate*, the challenge was ratcheted up: Everything had to follow the basic tenets of super-

clean eating as outlined by doctors—no loopholes—so that almost anyone with a food sensitivity or on nearly any cleanse could use the recipes for inspiration. And use them seamlessly—in a way that didn't put the focus on what was missing from their plate, but rather on what was there. Mostly, I was searching for food that tasted and felt as nourishing as it was healthy. Self-care and self-love have become overused words, but I don't think these feelings are present enough in the kitchen or when we're sitting down to eat. (I type this as I'm hurriedly eating a leftover salad at my desk, in front of my laptop, before my next meeting.) I never want to cook or eat something that feels like a compromise, like I'm saying "no" to what my body is craving.

What also makes this book different for me is that I developed recipes to work as part of six different week-long healing cleanses—each one anchored by a trusted health expert and tailored to support the body through a challenge that has been a roadblock in my life or in the lives of friends or family at one time or another. I think of these mini cleanses as gateways to the potency of nutrient-dense, whole foods. After the recipes, the doctors share their respective perspectives on tackling weight-loss resistance, dealing with heavy metals, giving our adrenals a break, resetting from Candida, getting proactive about cardiovascular health, and tapping into the ancient wisdom of Ayurveda. (In the next section, you'll see more on how these different targeted cleanses are broken down.)

Healthy and delicious are not mutually exclusive. The challenge of cleaning up a recipe is inherently enticing to me—whether I'm experimenting at home, trying to approximate something from a fast-food joint that my family is partial to, or in the goop test kitchen putting my own spin on John Legend's fried chicken wings. I hope you see a little bit of all that—healthy, delicious, fun—in every recipe that follows.

Love,

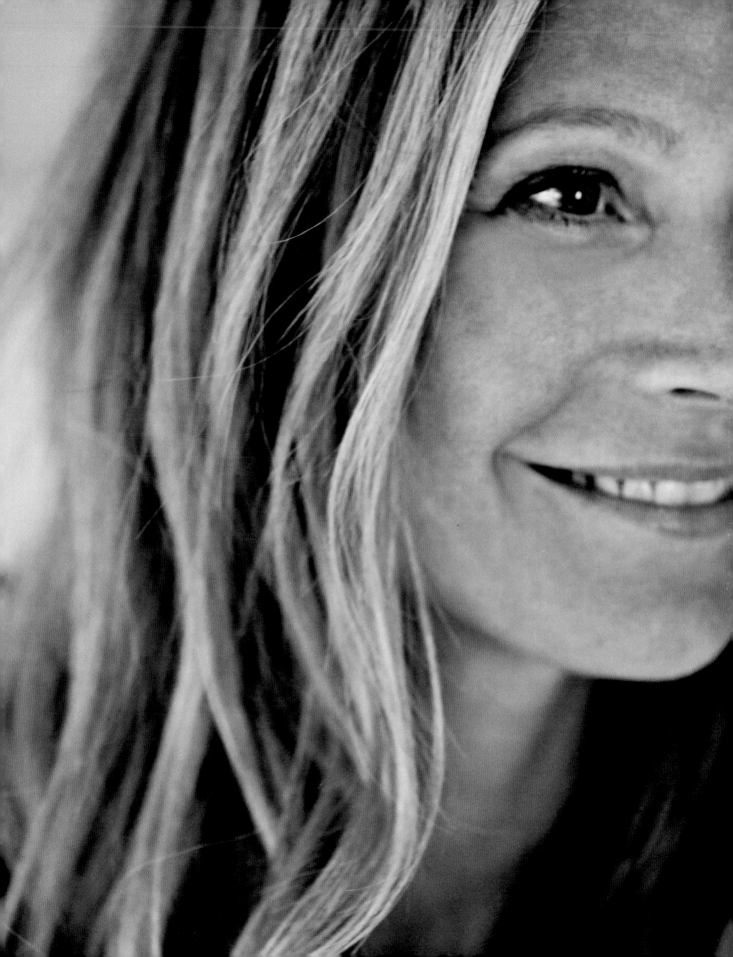

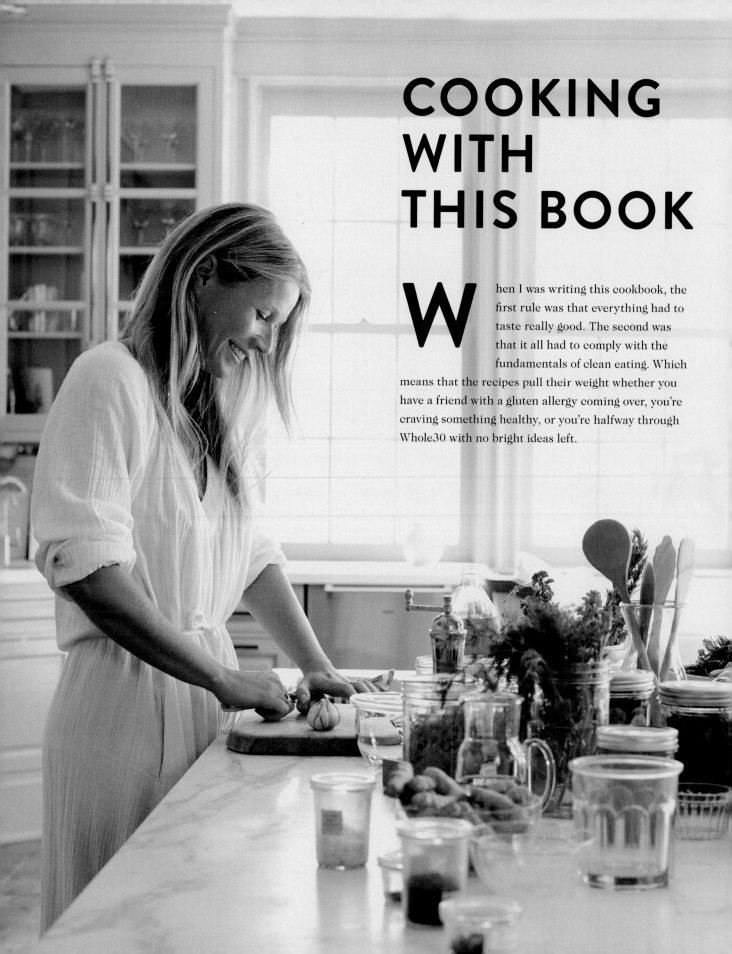

COOKING WITH THIS BOOK

When I was writing this cookbook, the first rule was that everything had to taste really good. The second was that it all had to comply with the fundamentals of clean eating. Which means that the recipes pull their weight whether you have a friend with a gluten allergy coming over, you're craving something healthy, or you're halfway through Whole30 with no bright ideas left.

Alcohol	Caffeine	Dairy
Gluten	Nightshades	Peanuts
Processed foods or sugars	Red meat	Soy

INSTEAD, YOU'LL FIND INGREDIENT SWAPS LIKE THESE:

Coconut aminos, a soy-free swap for tamari in marinades and dipping sauces.	Chickpea miso, for soy-free miso soups, marinades, and dressings.	Chickpea, lentil, or brown rice pasta as a gluten-free noodle fix.
Sugar-free kimchi (I like Wildbrine), which has all the flavor of regular kimchi and none of the typical added sugar.	Vanilla powder instead of vanilla extract, for alcohol-free, vanilla-flavored chia puddings and smoothies.	

Open to any recipe section any time you want a satisfying, nutritious meal. To make it easier to spot what you're after, you'll find three labels attributed to recipes throughout. (The threshold for "quick" here is under 30 minutes.)

PACKABLE

QUICK

VEGAN

A NOTE ON SERVING SIZES: The majority of the recipes in this book serve two, because when I'm cooking really clean, it's generally just for myself and leftovers. Most people aren't serving up completely clean meals for their families or at dinner parties. That said, my kids do like a bunch of the recipes in this book so I'll sometimes double certain recipes, and there are dishes you could liberally top off with Parmesan and butter to make them more appealing to

a crowd. You'll also see that some recipes are designed with bigger serving sizes in mind—particularly soups that wouldn't be worth it to make just one or two servings of, and which store/freeze well for later.

For those looking to go deeper into clean eating, in part II (page 215), I've put together six different menus, each good for a full week of clean eating, with a tailored twist. As mentioned in the introduction, these menus correspond to the slightly different food philosophies of six doctors, organized around varied health goals. Their respective takes on maximizing well-being are outlined in interviews with them that cover their lifestyle and detox recommendations beyond the kitchen. I also encourage you to look closer at their work, websites, and books, if they're relevant to what's going on in your personal health journey. And before following any protocol or plan, consult your own doctor to find out what's best and safe for you.

First up, beginning on page 217, is stabilizing metabolism and weight with Dr. Tasneem "Taz" Bhatia, a board-certified integrative medicine physician who combines both Western and Eastern medicine in her practice. Second (page 225) is getting rid of heavy metals with Dr. James Novak, whom I've come to know via Dr. Alejandro Junger. Dr. Junger spearheads his own chapter (page 231) on supporting your adrenal glands—akin to the outlet strip that your body plugs into for energy. The fourth targeted cleanse (page 237) is a specialty of Dr. Amy Myers, a functional medicine practitioner based in Austin, who has helped many patients rebalance their microbiomes after a Candida overgrowth. The fifth chapter (page 245) is with cardiologist turned nutrition expert Dr. Steven Gundry, who walks you through taking good care of your heart. Last is something for vegetarians or anyone in need of a plant-based diet: an accessible Ayurvedic cleanse (page 251), done in conjunction with leading Ayurveda expert Dr. Aruna Viswanathan.

PANTRY

Having a well-stocked pantry is one of the keys to cooking well at home. You might notice that the list of pantry items I used for *The Clean Plate* is shorter than the lists in my other cookbooks. That's because this is the cleanest I've ever had to cook. After cutting out so many processed foods and added sugars, I was left with nearly all raw ingredients. I've added an herbs and produce section because they are the most satisfying and nutritious ways to add flavor when cooking (and eating) clean. For produce, I aim for organic to avoid pesticides and herbicides that are typically sprayed on conventional fruits and veggies.

Last, beans are a favorite non-meat source of protein. If you are trying to avoid lectins (see Dr. Gundry's explanation of this plant protein on page 247), beans should be pressure cooked, which gets rid of the lectins. I either do this myself at home, or buy Eden Foods brand canned beans, which are pressure cooked (most canned beans aren't).

OILS, VINEGARS, AND SAUCES

Apple cider vinegar

Coconut aminos

Coconut oil

Extra virgin olive oil

Good-quality fish sauce, like Red Boat

Sunflower seed oil

Tahini

Toasted sesame oil

CANNED GOODS

Anchovies

Beans (Eden Foods)

Capers

RICES, PASTAS, FLOURS, AND OTHER PANTRY ITEMS

Brown, black, and basmati rice

Buckwheat groats

Chia seeds

Chickpea flour

Chickpea, lentil, or brown rice pasta

Flaxseed

Millet

Nori sheets

Quinoa

Raw nuts and seeds like cashews, almonds, pepitas (pumpkin seeds), and sunflower and sesame seeds

FOR SWEETNESS

Almond butter

Dates

Liquid stevia (not stevia-based sweeteners)

Raw cacao powder

Unsweetened shredded coconut

SPICES

Aleppo pepper

Bay leaves

Black pepper

Cardamom

Chili flakes

Cinnamon

Coriander

Cumin

Curry powder

Garam masala

Kosher salt

Maldon sea salt

Mexican oregano

Turmeric

Za'atar

FRESH HERBS AND PRODUCE

Basil

Chives

Cilantro

Garlic

Ginger

Leeks

Lemons and limes

Mint

Parsley

Red, white, and yellow onions

Rosemary

Scallions

Tarragon

Thyme

SOME ESSENTIAL TOOLS

Food processor

Immersion blender

Mandoline

Microplane rasp grater

Spiralizer

Vitamix blender

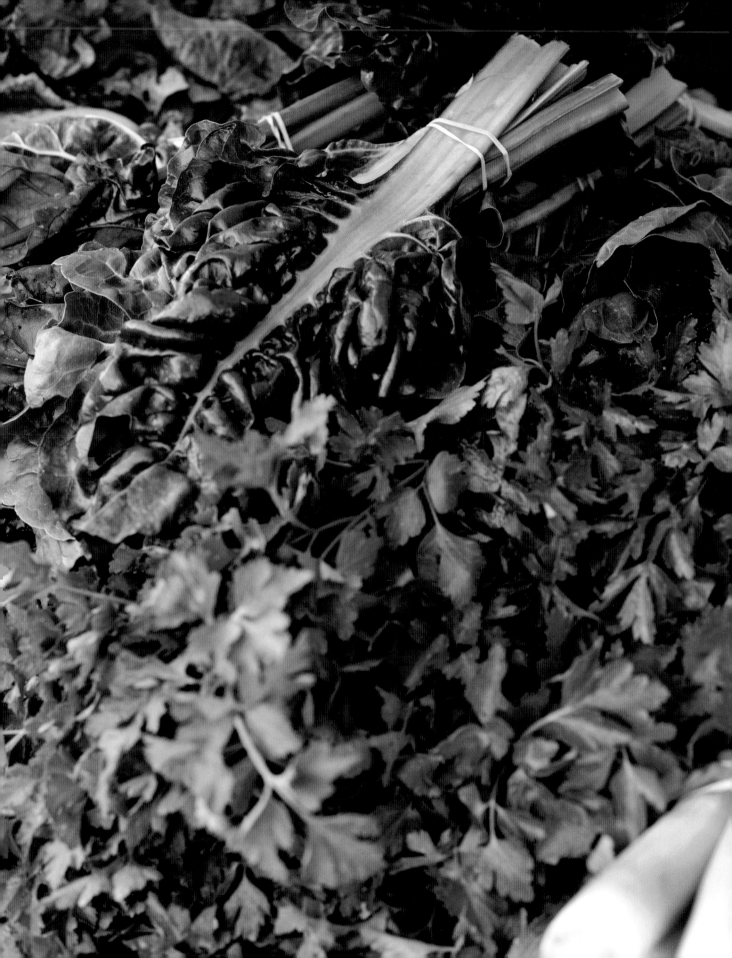

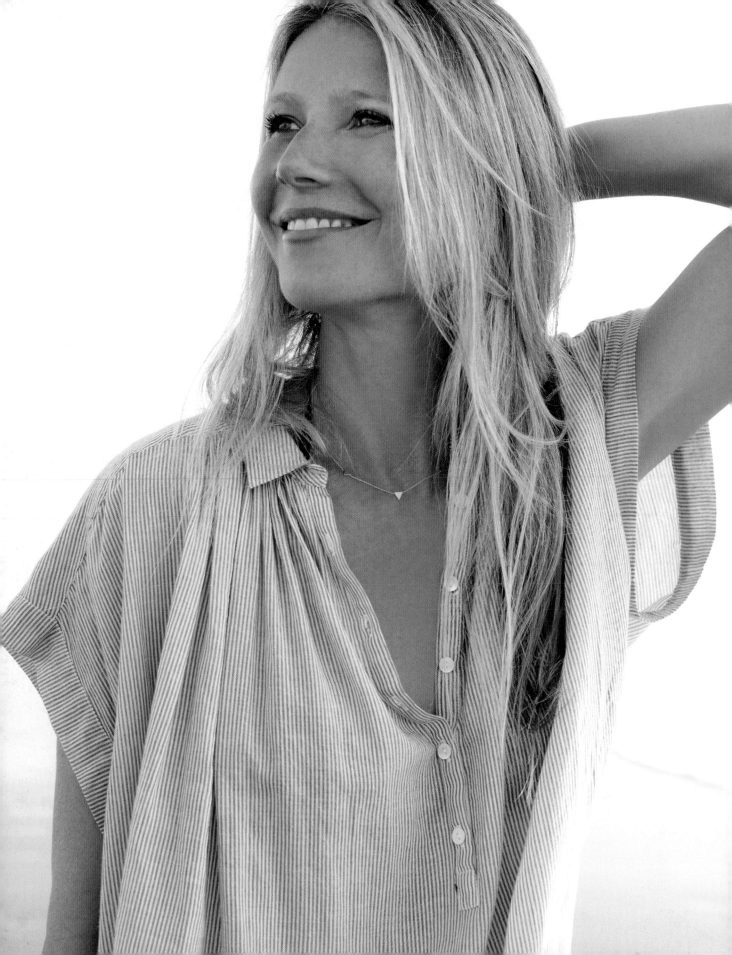

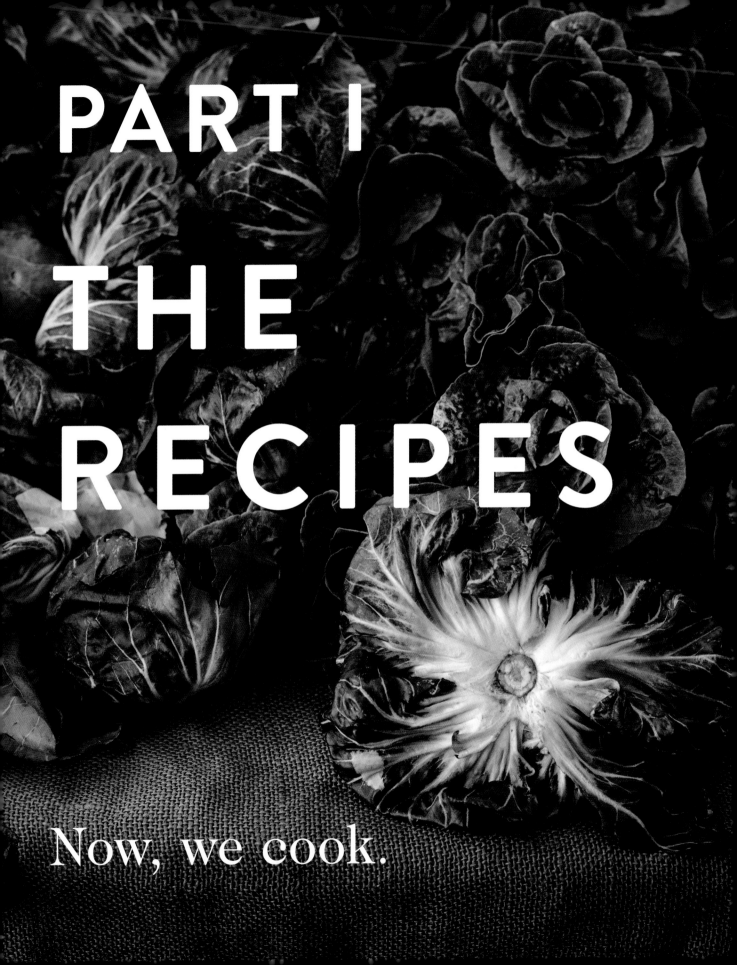

PART I

THE

RECIPES

Now, we cook.

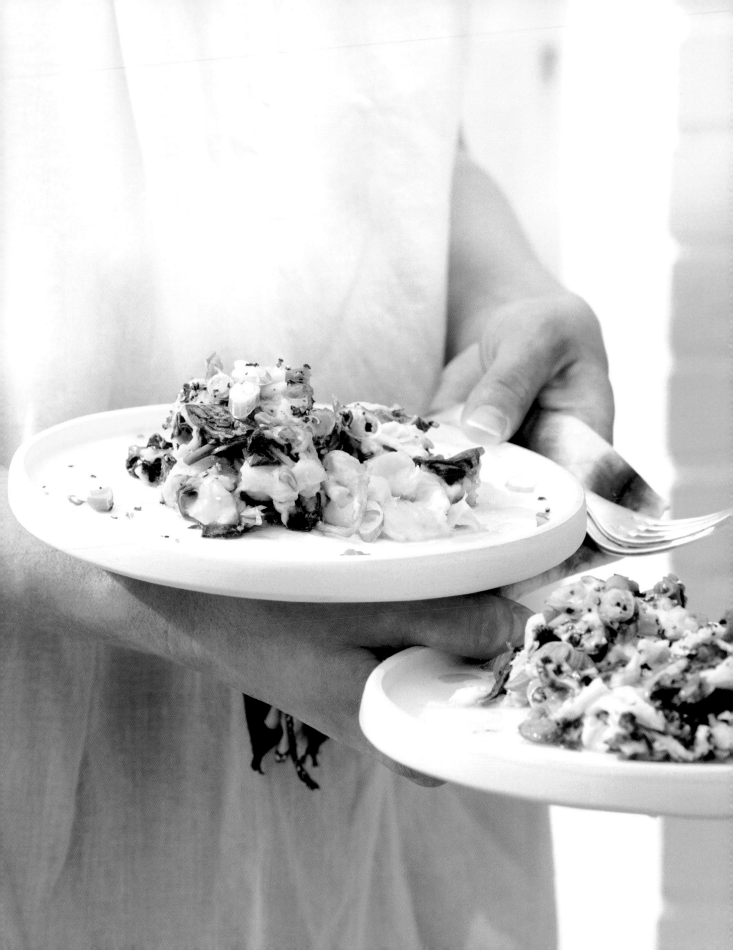

BREAKFAST

With its morning buns, chocolate croissants, and fruit juices, breakfast is a minefield of sugar and empty calories, which can amp you up, then leave you crashed and in recovery mode by ten a.m. Not exactly the best way to start your day on the regular. Plus, if you lean toward the savory side like me, these conventional offerings aren't all that appealing or satisfying. Most weekday mornings, I actually opt for an easy smoothie that's light on the sugar (see the drinks chapter on page 149), but when I'm cooking breakfast—which is generally weekend brunch with family—I like to try for dishes that can keep you full until lunchtime. With a little planning (and some key ingredients), a quick and seriously nutritious breakfast—like black rice pudding with mango, chocolate milk chia pudding, or dal with sautéed chard—is right at your fingertips. Because I know not everyone shares my affinity for savory at all times of the day, I layered in ingredients for the sweet-toothed among us. Whether you're after quick-and-easy weekday inspiration or a brunch-worthy dish, this mix of recipes has you covered.

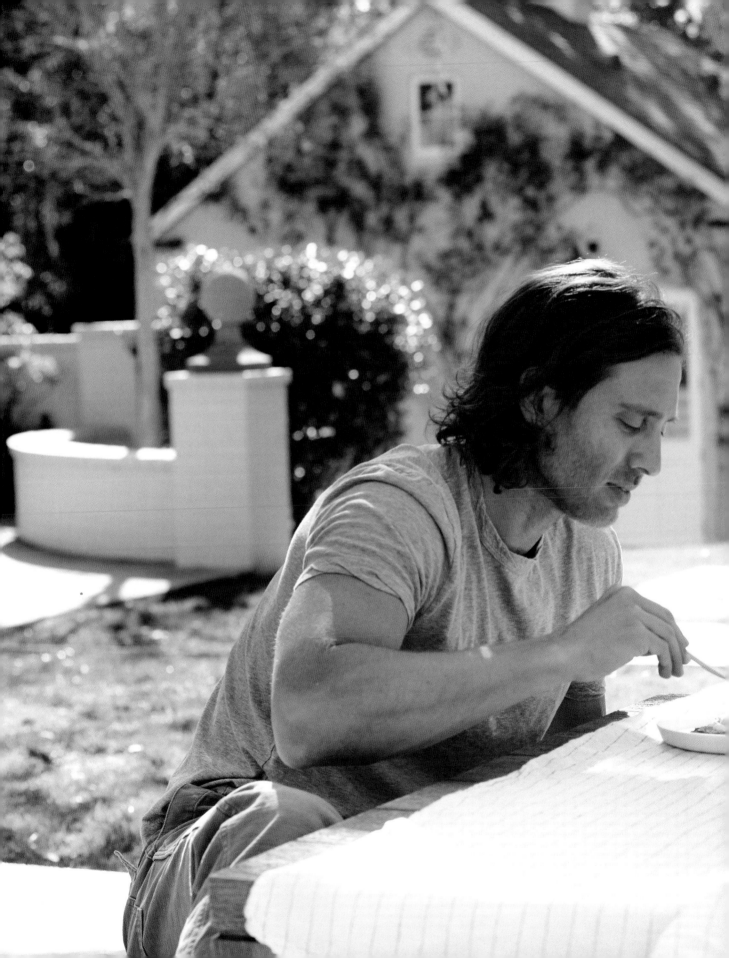

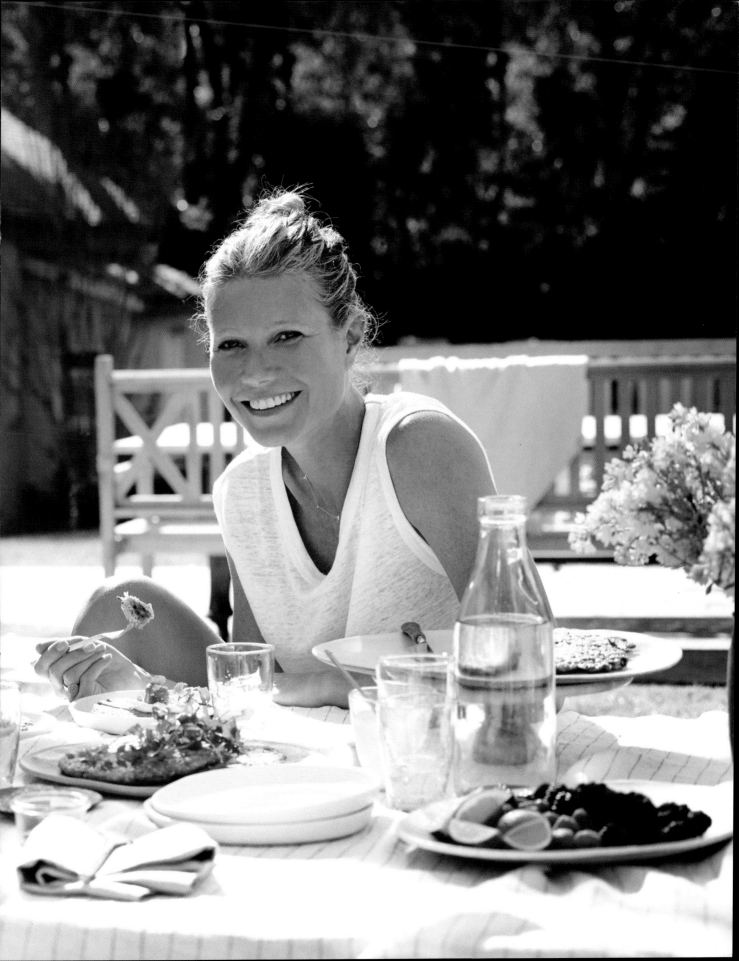

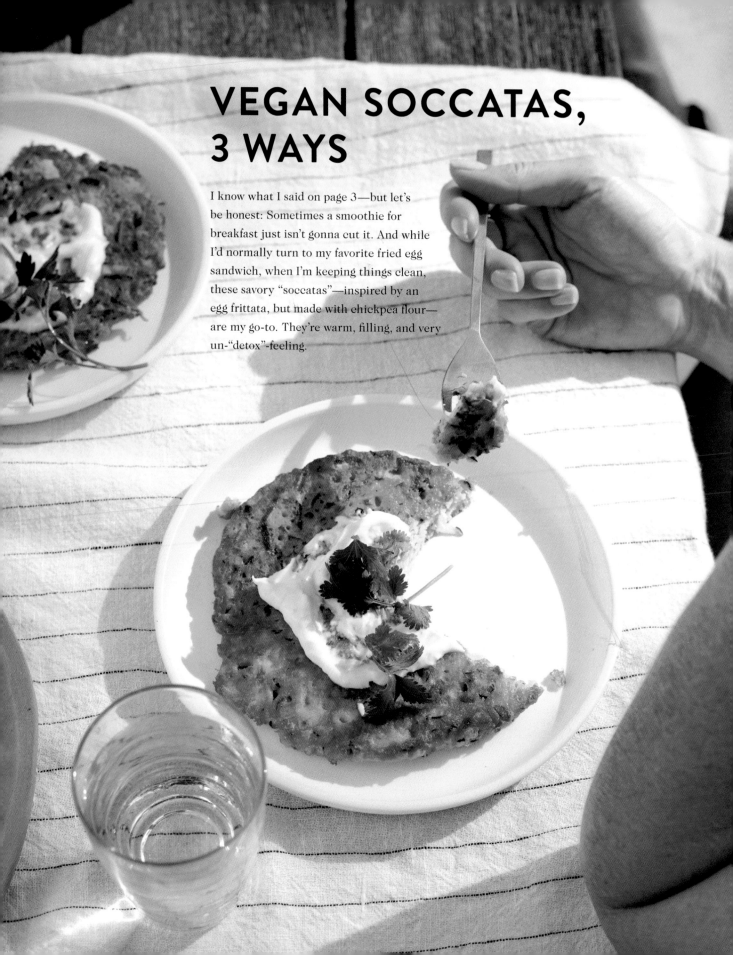

VEGAN SOCCATAS, 3 WAYS

I know what I said on page 3—but let's be honest: Sometimes a smoothie for breakfast just isn't gonna cut it. And while I'd normally turn to my favorite fried egg sandwich, when I'm keeping things clean, these savory "soccatas"—inspired by an egg frittata, but made with chickpea flour—are my go-to. They're warm, filling, and very un-"detox"-feeling.

Cauliflower, Pea & Turmeric Soccata

VEGAN

Serves 2

My kids are crazy for samosas, stuffed with cauliflower, peas, and potatoes and served with a mint or cilantro chutney. I used those flavors as inspiration here, filling the soccata with cauliflower and peas (skipping the potatoes to keep it nightshade-free) and topping it with a fresh herb salad. These make an elegant brunch option, but are also nice for lunch or dinner.

½ cup chickpea flour

½ cup water

2 teaspoons olive oil, plus more as needed

½ teaspoon kosher salt

⅔ cup steamed cauliflower florets (I use frozen organic cauliflower)

⅔ cup frozen peas

1 teaspoon grated lime zest

2 scallions, thinly sliced

½ teaspoon ground turmeric

2 tablespoons fresh cilantro leaves

2 tablespoons torn fresh mint leaves

2 tablespoons fresh parsley leaves

Juice of ½ lime

Flaky sea salt

½ ripe avocado, thinly sliced (optional)

In a medium bowl, whisk together the chickpea flour, water, olive oil, and kosher salt.

Add the cauliflower florets, mashing them a bit with a fork. Stir in the peas, lime zest, scallions, and turmeric.

Heat an 8-inch nonstick skillet over medium-high heat. Add about 1 tablespoon olive oil, and pour in half the batter. Cook for about 4 minutes, or until the bottom is starting to crisp, then flip the pancake and cook for 3 minutes or so on the second side.

Transfer the soccata to a plate and cook the second soccata.

In a small bowl, toss the cilantro, mint, and parsley with the lime juice, a little olive oil, and a pinch of flaky salt.

Top each soccata with some sliced avocado, if desired, and garnish with the herb salad.

Kale Kuku Soccata

VEGAN

Serves 2

Inspired by the Persian egg dish *kuku*, this vegan *kuku* gets a healthy dose of sliced kale in addition to the typical fresh herbs.

¾ cup chickpea flour

¾ cup water

1 tablespoon olive oil, plus more as needed

¾ teaspoon kosher salt

1⅓ cups thinly sliced kale leaves

2 tablespoons minced fresh parsley

2 tablespoons minced fresh dill

2 tablespoons minced fresh cilantro

2 scallions, thinly sliced

1 teaspoon grated lemon zest

Lemony Garlic Aquafaba Sauce (page 179; optional)

½ ripe avocado, thinly sliced (optional)

In a medium bowl, whisk together the chickpea flour, water, olive oil, and kosher salt.

Stir in the kale, parsley, dill, cilantro, scallions, and lemon zest.

Heat an 8-inch nonstick skillet over medium-high heat. Add about 1 tablespoon olive oil, and pour in half the batter. Cook for about 4 minutes, or until the bottom is starting to crisp, then flip the pancake and cook for 3 minutes or so on the second side.

Transfer the soccata to a plate and cook the second soccata.

Serve with a dollop of lemony garlic aquafaba and garnish with avocado, if desired.

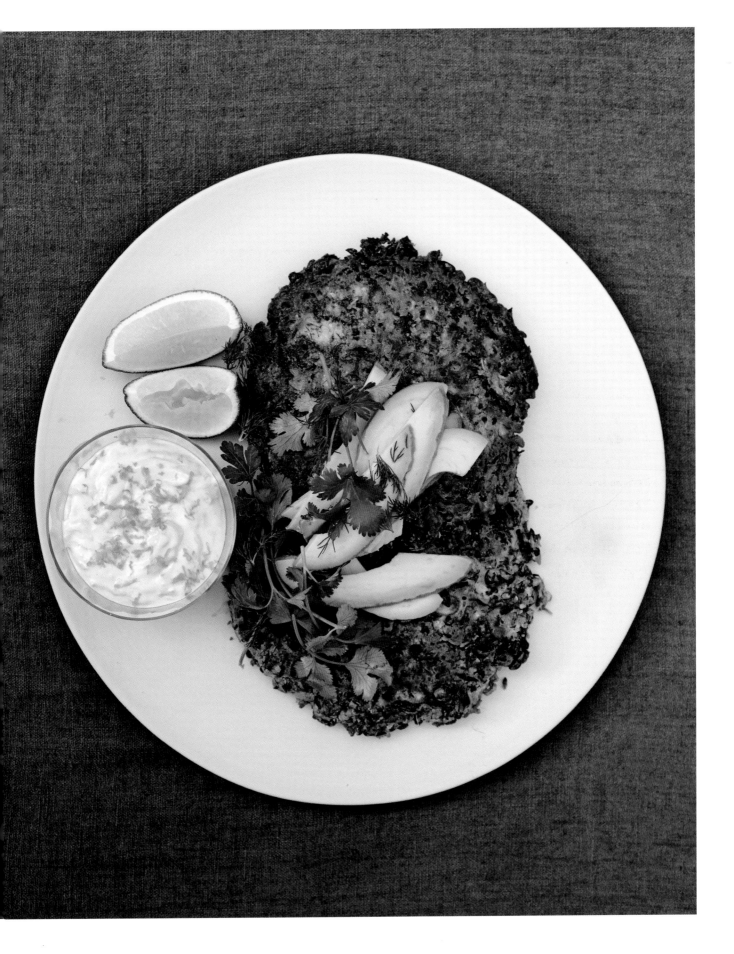

Zucchini & Lemon Soccata

VEGAN

Serves 2

Zucchini contains a lot of water, so make this batter right before you plan to cook it. Otherwise, the zucchini can make the mixture too watery.

½ cup chickpea flour

½ cup water

2 teaspoons olive oil, plus more as needed

½ teaspoon kosher salt

1⅓ cups grated zucchini (about 1 zucchini)

1 teaspoon grated lemon zest

2 scallions, thinly sliced

A large pinch of Aleppo pepper (optional)

In a medium bowl, whisk together the chickpea flour, water, olive oil, and kosher salt.

Stir in the zucchini, lemon zest, scallion, and Aleppo pepper (if using).

Heat an 8-inch nonstick skillet over medium-high heat. Add about 1 tablespoon olive oil, and pour in half the batter. Cook for about 4 minutes, or until the bottom is starting to crisp, then flip the pancake and cook for 3 minutes or so on the second side.

Transfer the soccata to a plate and cook the second soccata.

Breakfast Dal

VEGAN

Serves 2

This warming, savory breakfast is both easy and satisfying (and would be delicious at any time of day). I love the chard here, as it's a not-too-hearty, not-too-delicate green, but any greens you have on hand will do in a pinch.

1 tablespoon coconut oil, plus more if needed

½ white or yellow onion, finely diced

Scant ½ teaspoon kosher salt

1 tablespoon curry powder

½ teaspoon grated fresh ginger

½ cup red lentils

1½ cups water

½ cup torn Swiss chard leaves

In a small saucepan, melt the coconut oil over medium heat. Add the onion and salt and cook, stirring, until softened, 3 to 5 minutes. Add the curry powder and ginger, stir, and cook for a couple of minutes more, until very fragrant. Add the lentils and water. Cook, stirring frequently, for 8 to 10 minutes, until the lentils are tender and the dal is thick, adding additional water if needed to get the desired consistency.

In a small skillet, melt about 1 teaspoon of coconut oil over medium-high heat. Add the Swiss chard and cook, stirring, until tender, for 3 minutes. Alternatively, simply stir the chard directly into the dal and let it gently cook.

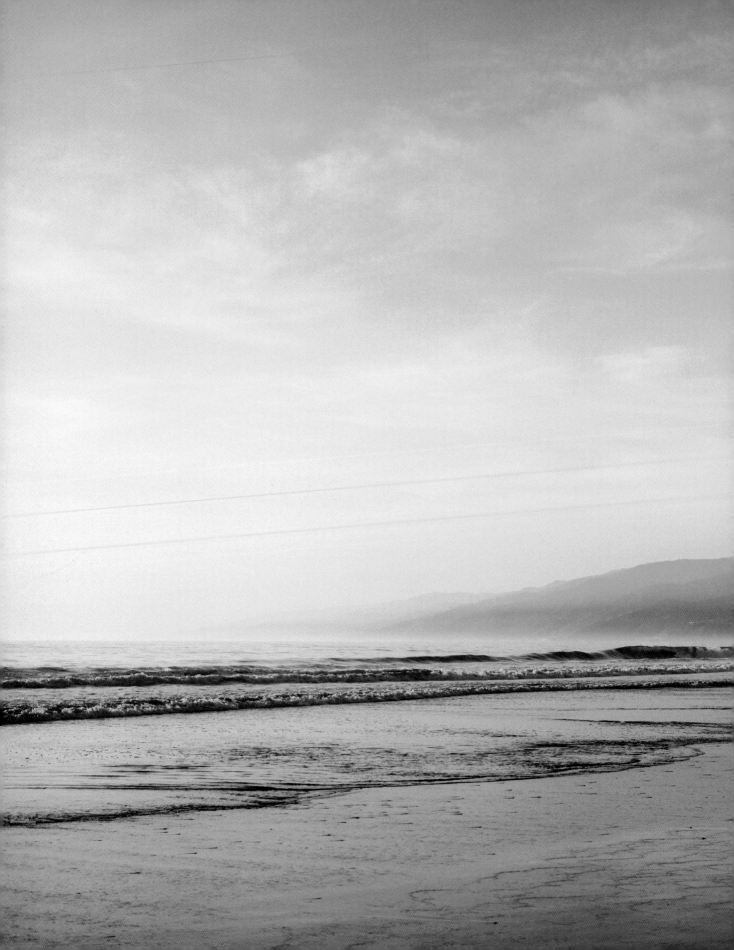

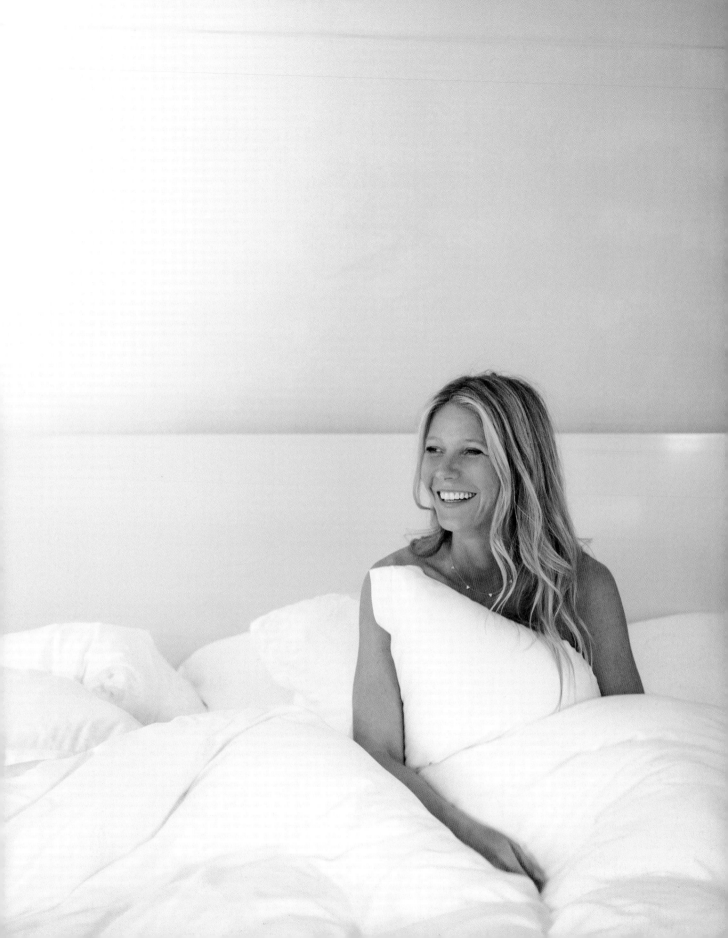

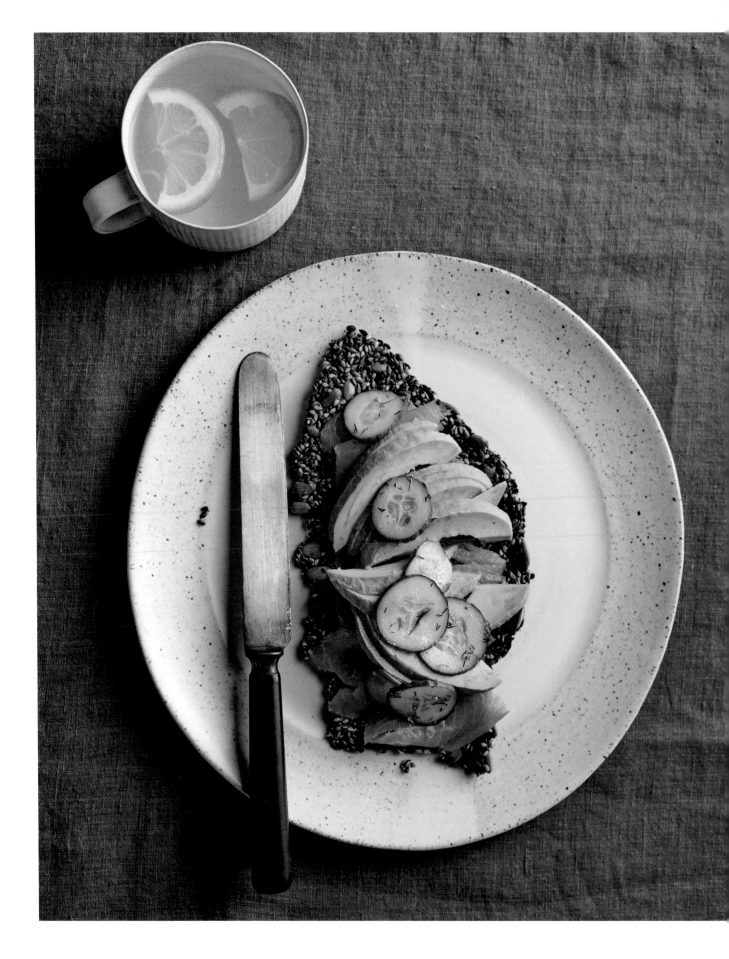

Seed Cracker with Smoked Salmon & Avocado

Serves 2

Once your cracker is made, this no-brainer breakfast—full of skin-friendly omega-3s—is so quick and easy to throw together. While the cracker recipe was inspired by chef Magnus Nilsson, I made this variation with Dr. Taz Bhatia in mind—see page 220 where she explains how healthy fats help balance insulin, keep blood sugar levels stable, and make you feel satiated. If you have a Microplane, grate a little fresh lemon zest over the salmon here while you're at it.

2 large pieces Seed Cracker (page 203)

2 ounces good-quality smoked salmon

1 avocado, thinly sliced

Pickled Cucumbers (page 209)

Fresh lemon juice

Flaky sea salt and cracked black pepper

Top the crackers with the smoked salmon, avocado, and a few pickled cucumbers.

Squeeze lemon juice over the top and sprinkle with a little flaky salt and cracked pepper.

Seed Cracker with Egg & Avocado

Serves 2

Instead of forgoing avocado toast altogether—which can be tough for some people to digest—when eliminating gluten and grains, I sub in a seed cracker for the toast. This one gets topped with a boiled egg for a little extra protein, but feel free to skip it if you're not eating eggs (I'm not sensitive to them, but I know others can be) and/or you want to keep things vegan.

2 large eggs

2 large pieces Seed Cracker (page 203)

1 small avocado, thinly sliced

Flaky sea salt and cracked black pepper

Pickled Red Onions (page 206)

Bring a small saucepan of water to a boil. Add the eggs and set a timer for 8 minutes. Meanwhile, fill a medium bowl with ice and water. When the timer goes off, use a slotted spoon to plunge the eggs into the ice bath and let cool. When they're cool enough to handle, peel and slice the eggs.

Top the crackers with avocado and egg. Season with flaky salt and cracked pepper, and garnish with a few pickled onions.

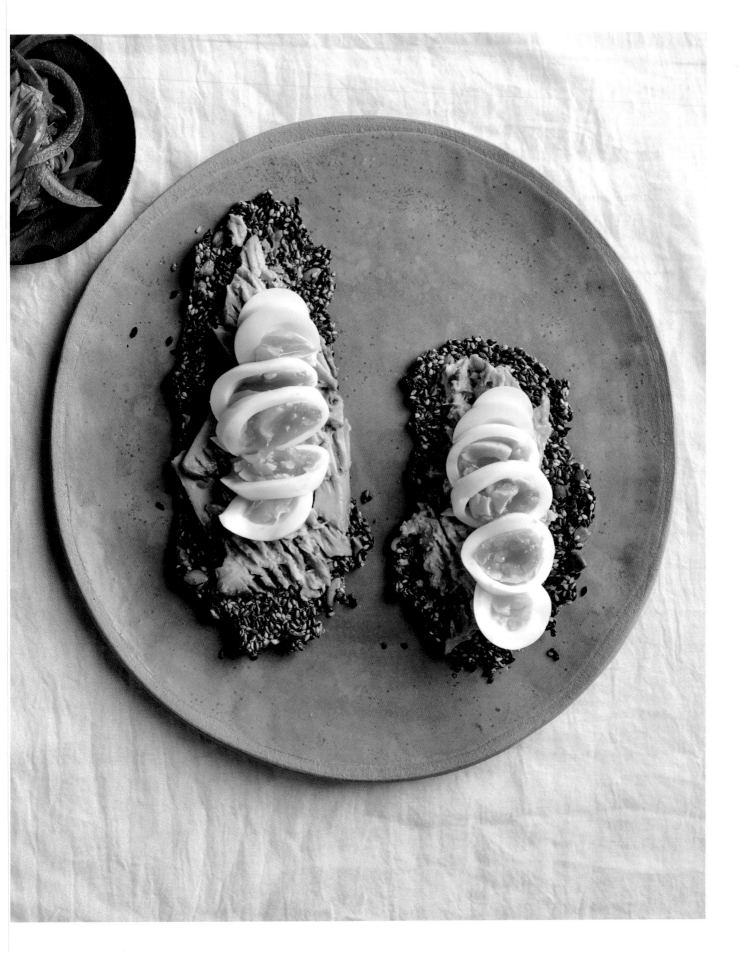

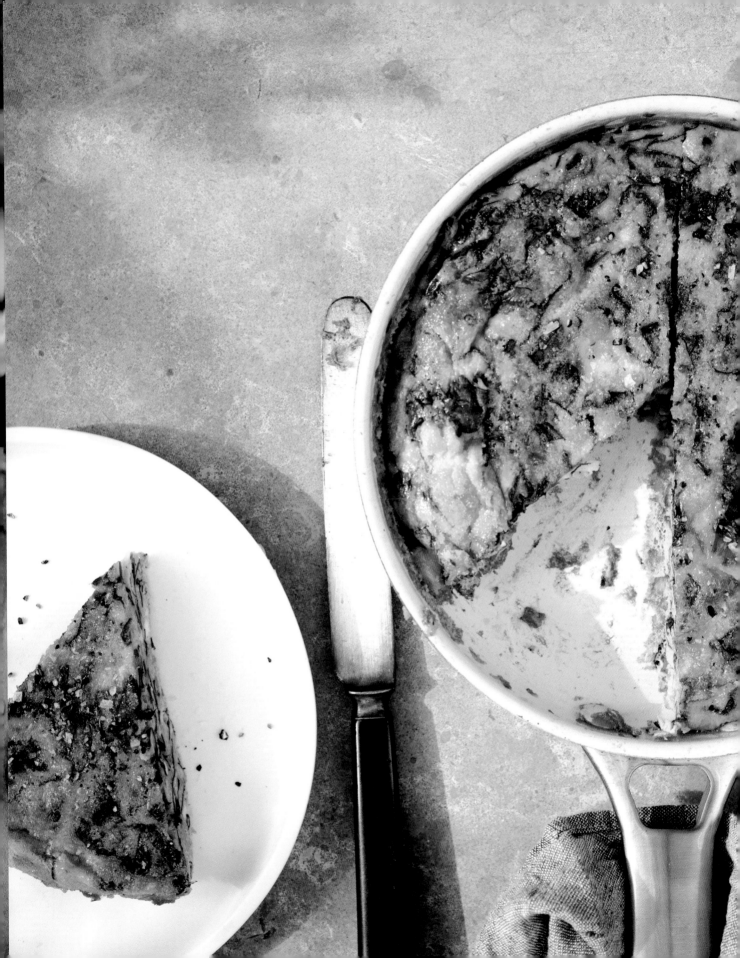

Easy Frittata

QUICK

Serves 2

Frittatas are perfect for using up veggie scraps. When testing recipes for this book, I used a lot of beets (beets and I were having a moment), so I always had leftover beet greens around the kitchen. I tried adding them to a frittata with some shallots, and it was a hit.

2 tablespoons olive oil

¼ cup diced shallots

1½ to 2 cups chopped beet greens

Kosher salt and freshly ground black pepper

4 large eggs, beaten

Preheat the oven to 375°F.

In an 8-inch oven-safe nonstick skillet, heat the olive oil over medium-high heat. Add the shallots and cook, stirring, for a couple of minutes, until softened, then stir in the beet greens and cook until wilted. Season with a generous pinch each of salt and pepper. Add the eggs and turn off the heat. Pop the skillet in the oven for about 10 minutes, or until the eggs are set.

Slice and serve.

Poached Eggs over Sautéed Greens

QUICK

Serves 2

Runny egg yolk and sautéed greens are a match made in heaven. I know people claim you need vinegar to properly poach an egg, but I'm not buying it. Just be sure to keep the water vortex moving by stirring gently but consistently as the eggs cook at a nice, low simmer.

2 tablespoons olive oil

⅓ cup thinly sliced leeks

Heaping 1½ cups chopped chard leaves

Kosher salt

2 large eggs

Freshly ground black pepper

Bring a large saucepan of water to a simmer.

Meanwhile, in a medium nonstick skillet, heat the olive oil over medium-low heat. Add the leeks and cook for 3 minutes, then stir in the chard and a large pinch of salt.

Crack the eggs into small ramekins and add them one at a time to the simmering water, using a large slotted spoon to carefully make sure they are not sticking to the bottom of the saucepan. Cook for 2½ minutes, or until the white is fully cooked but the yolk still feels tender when gently pressed with a fingertip.

Divide the greens between two plates, top each with a poached egg, and sprinkle with salt and pepper.

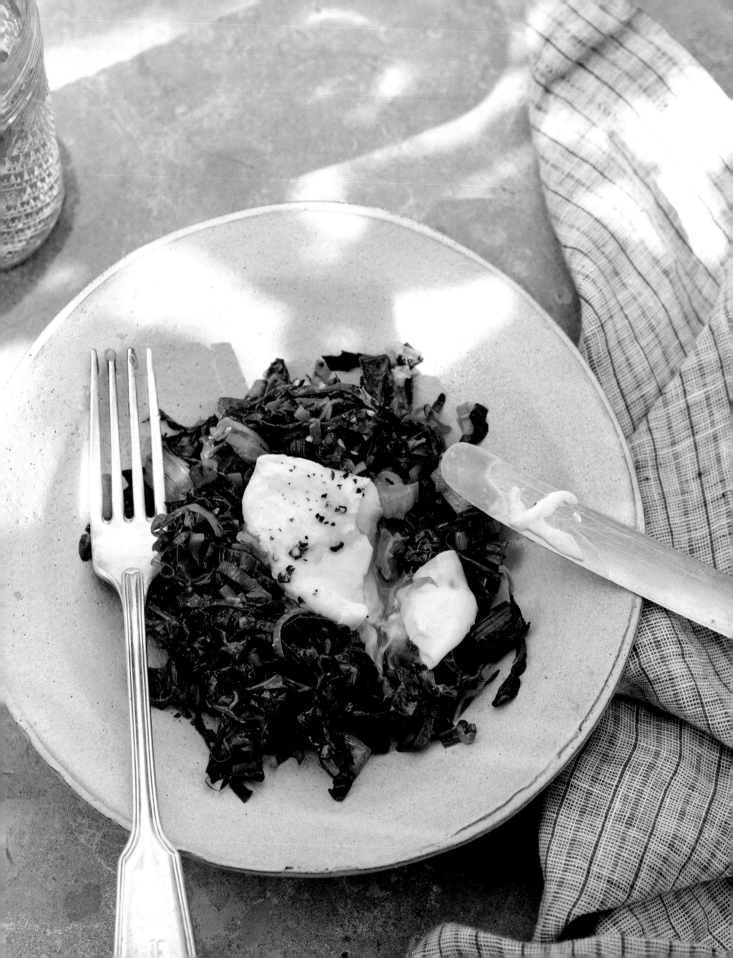

Quinoa Cereal with Freeze-Dried Berries

VEGAN

Serves 2

My daughter loves freeze-dried berries, and they are so tasty in cereal that I thought I'd try a homemade cereal for a lighter breakfast option. My local co-op's bulk bin had nutty puffed quinoa crisps—akin to detox Rice Krispies. This recipe makes enough for two servings, but you could scale the recipe up and store it in a mason jar to have all week long.

1 cup quinoa crisps

¼ cup freeze-dried blueberries

¼ cup freeze-dried raspberries

¼ cup toasted sunflower seeds

¼ teaspoon ground cinnamon

A pinch of flaky sea salt

Nondairy milk, for serving

Combine all the ingredients in a medium bowl. Divide between two serving bowls and serve with your (alternative) milk of choice. Store any leftover dry cereal mix in an airtight container at room temperature for up to 2 weeks.

Sweet Buckwheat Porridge

VEGAN

Serves 2

For a lazy morning at home—of which there are not nearly enough—I turn to a warm, cozy porridge, and buckwheat makes for a great gluten-free alternative. If brown sugar is part of your normal oatmeal routine, I think you'll be surprised how well the dates and apples sub in for sweetness. Personally, I just love the texture of the groats in contrast to the juicy, crisp apple.

½ cup buckwheat groats, soaked overnight in water

1 cup unsweetened almond milk

1 date, pitted and chopped

1 tablespoon unsweetened almond butter

½ Granny Smith apple, cored and diced

¼ teaspoon ground cinnamon or cloves

Flaky sea salt

Drain the soaked groats and put them in a small saucepan. Add the almond milk and date and bring to a boil. Reduce the heat to low, cover, and cook for 10 to 15 minutes. Stir in the almond butter and apple.

Divide between two bowls, sprinkle with the cinnamon and flaky salt, and serve.

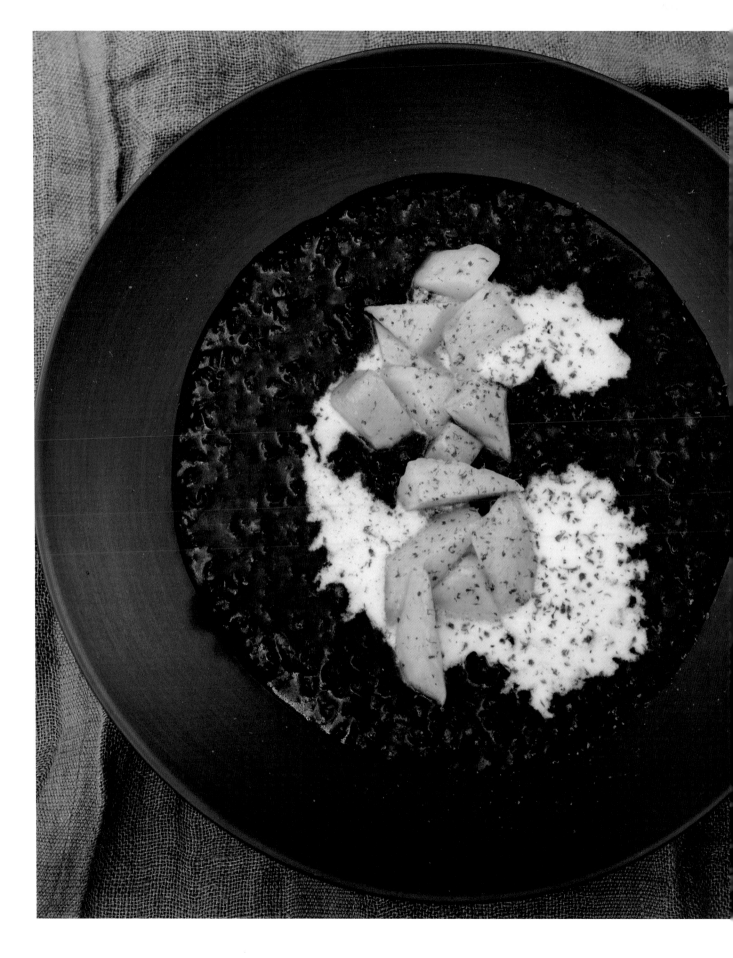

Black Rice Pudding with Coconut Milk & Mango

VEGAN

Serves 2

Full of iron, vitamin E, and antioxidants, black rice is a nutritional powerhouse. It also happens to be delicious. Here I simmer it slowly in water and coconut milk, and top it with ripe mango. It plays to both sides—a little sweet, a little salty. In the right crowd, I'd even get away with serving it for dessert.

½ cup black rice

2 cups water

½ cup plus 2 tablespoons full-fat coconut milk

1 date, pitted and diced

¼ teaspoon kosher salt

½ mango, peeled and sliced

In a small saucepan, combine the rice, water, ½ cup of the coconut milk, the date, and the salt. Bring to a boil, then reduce the heat to maintain a simmer, cover, and cook for 45 minutes, stirring halfway through to make sure the rice is not sticking.

Divide the rice pudding between two bowls and pour 1 tablespoon of the coconut milk over each. Top with the mango and serve.

Chocolate Chia Pudding

PACKABLE / QUICK / VEGAN

Serves 2

I like to think of this as a healthy, grown-up version of the "snack pack"–style chocolate pudding I grew up with as a kid. This was designed for breakfast, but also works well as an afternoon pick-me-up if you have a sweet tooth. Plus, it's a great way to get antioxidant-rich superfoods like maca (which I've been told by doctors and nutritionists alike is particularly good for sexual health) into your diet.

2 cups full-fat coconut milk

½ cup water

1 tablespoon raw cacao powder

2 teaspoons maca (optional)

4 dates, pitted and finely chopped

½ teaspoon kosher salt

⅛ teaspoon vanilla powder (optional)

½ cup chia seeds

Cacao nibs, to garnish (optional)

In a medium bowl, whisk together the coconut milk, water, cacao powder, maca (if using), dates, salt, and vanilla (if using) until well combined.

Whisk in the chia seeds and let sit at room temperature for 5 minutes, stirring every minute or so to make sure the seeds are evenly mixed.

Eat immediately, garnished with cacao nibs, if desired, or cover and store in the fridge for up to 4 days.

Beet Açai Blueberry Smoothie Bowl

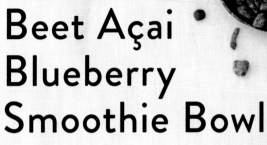
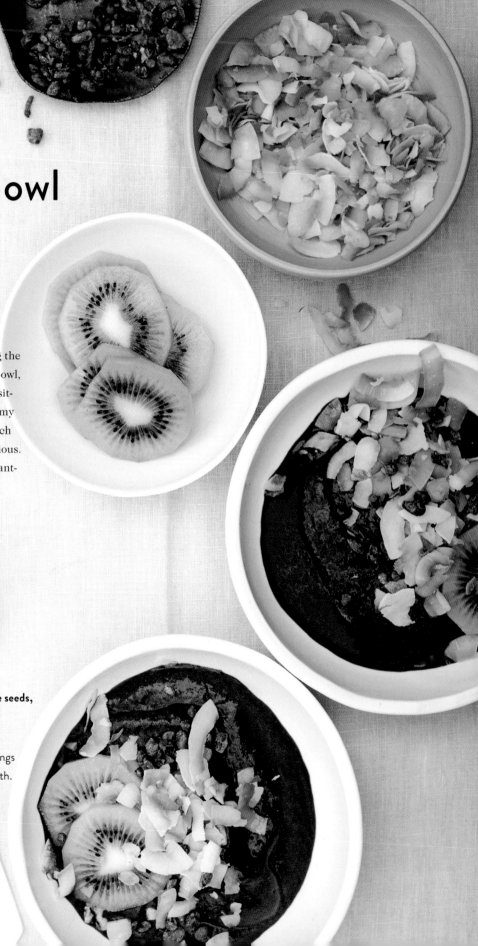

QUICK / VEGAN

Serves 2

Sometimes I'm burnt out on "drinking" breakfast even if I'm actually still craving the taste of a smoothie. Enter the smoothie bowl, which can add a bit more ceremony to a sit-down breakfast, even if it's happening at my desk during a meeting with the goop merch team. This one is as colorful as it is delicious. Not to mention, it's packed with antioxidant-rich beets, açai, and blueberries.

¼ cup chopped Roasted Beets (page 198)

2 (5-ounce) packs frozen açai

½ cup full-fat coconut milk

½ cup coconut water

½ cup frozen blueberries

Scant ¼ teaspoon ground cardamom

Zest and juice of 1 lime

Suggested toppings: toasted coconut flakes, Quinoa Cereal (page 24), kiwi, pomegranate seeds, cacao nibs

Combine all the ingredients except the toppings in a high-speed blender and blend until smooth. Pour into small bowls and garnish with your toppings of choice.

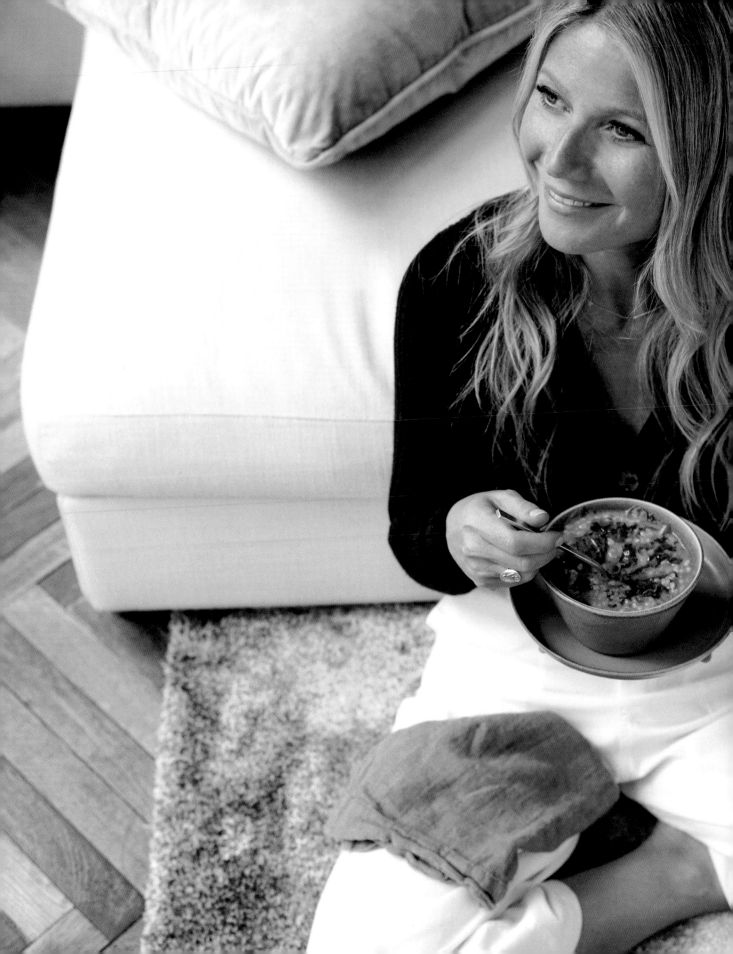

SOUPS

I can't think of anything more comforting than a bowl of soup. I leaned on soups hard to warm me up when I lived in chillier London, but they're a big part of my cooking repertoire in sunnier LA, too. I still get nostalgic for chicken soup—all the women on the Jewish side of my family had their own divine recipes— particularly when I'm feeling not so great. As far as clean eating goes, soups are traditionally made from vegetables, bone broth, and other inherently good-for-you ingredients, so they're usually in line with whatever detox-esque regimen I come across in my wellness deep dives or get asked to guinea pig by the goop edit girls. They rarely need much (if any) tweaking. And because my entire family will happily eat them, I've almost always got a Dutch oven of something soupy simmering on the stove and a stockpile of favorites in the freezer. Packed with home runs like bright and brothy pho, the stickiest turmeric rice porridge, and a refreshing cucumber-avocado gazpacho, this chapter has a soup for every palate, season, and hunger level.

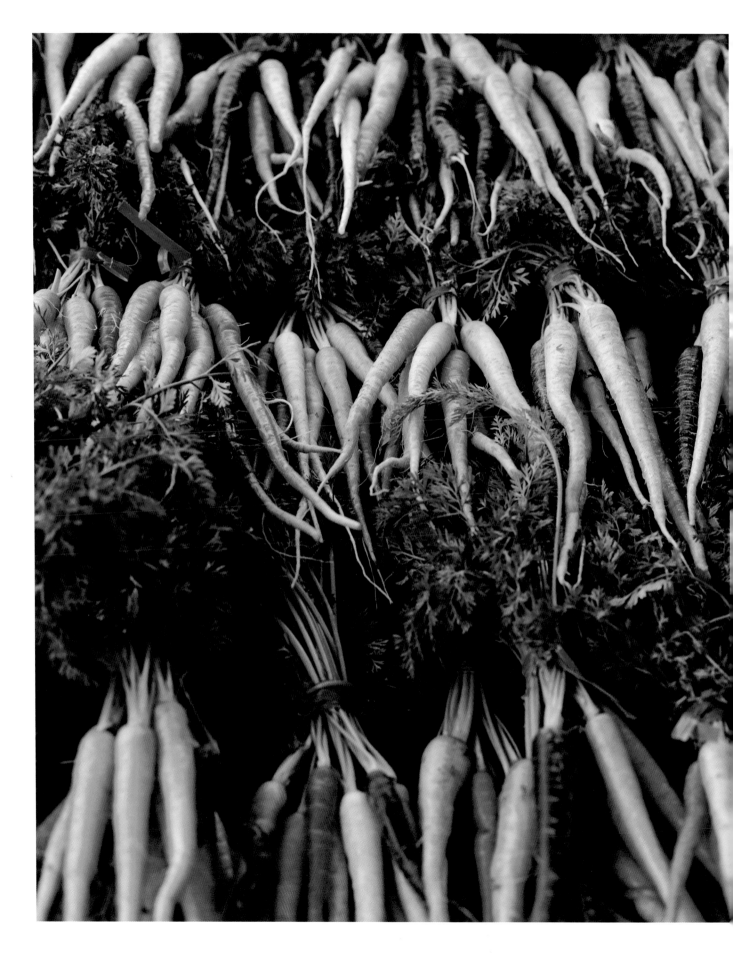

Clean Carrot Soup

Serves 4

An oldie but a goodie, I've been cooking this carrot soup for years. Made with just five ingredients (not including the olive oil, salt, and pepper), it's so simple to put together, but still seriously delivers in the flavor department.

6 to 8 medium to large carrots (about 1½ pounds), diced into rustic cubes

Flaky sea salt and freshly ground black pepper

3 tablespoons olive oil, plus more as needed

6 cups Chicken Stock or Vegetable Stock (pages 193 and 192)

1 (1-inch) piece fresh ginger, peeled

1 small white or yellow onion, chopped

2 garlic cloves

Preheat the oven to 375°F.

Place half the carrots on a baking sheet. Season with salt and pepper and drizzle lightly with olive oil. Toss to combine. Bake for about 20 minutes, shaking the pan every so often for even cooking, until soft, lightly browned, and caramelized. Remove from the oven.

Meanwhile, in a large saucepan, combine the stock, ginger, onion, and garlic. Bring to a boil, then reduce the heat to maintain a simmer and cook for about 5 minutes, or until the onions are soft. Add the raw carrots and simmer for 5 minutes, until the carrots are just slightly soft but not cooked through.

Carefully transfer the mixture to a blender, add the roasted carrots, and blend until smooth (work in batches, if necessary, and be careful when blending hot liquids). Alternatively, add the roasted carrots to the saucepan and blend the soup directly in the pan with an immersion blender.

To serve, pour or ladle into bowls, season with salt and pepper, and add a drizzle of olive oil over each portion.

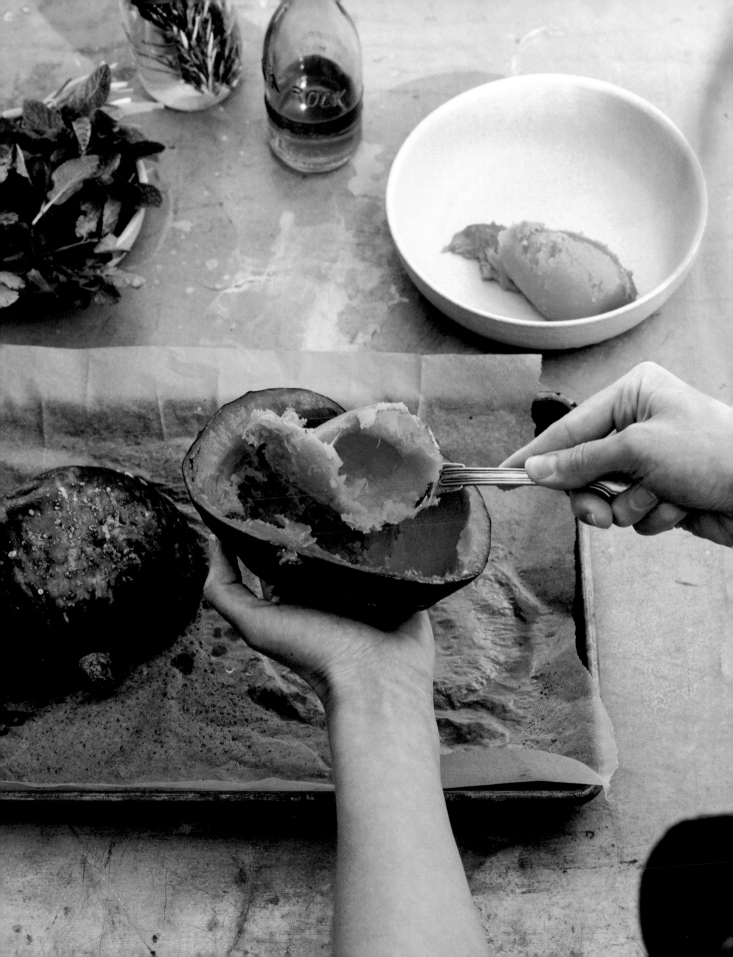

Roasted Kabocha Soup

VEGAN

Serves 4

Thanks to its inherent starchiness, kabocha—an orange-fleshed Japanese squash—makes the most incredible creamy, dairy-free soups. This recipe only uses half of one squash, but I always roast the whole thing and throw the other half into grain bowls and salads throughout the week. (P.S. If you've heard of lectins—a plant-based protein that Dr. Gundry recommends his patients with autoimmunity and cardiovascular concerns limit—and you want to try cutting them out, you can do so by seeding and peeling seeded veggies like squash. For more, see page 247.)

½ medium kabocha squash, seeded

Kosher salt and freshly ground black pepper

2 tablespoons olive oil

2 tablespoons coconut oil

1 large onion, sliced

2 garlic cloves, sliced

2 tablespoons chopped fresh ginger

1 teaspoon ground cumin

½ teaspoon ground coriander

½ teaspoon garam masala

3 cups Vegetable Stock (page 192)

Preheat the oven to 400°F. Line a baking sheet with parchment paper.

Season the squash generously with salt and pepper, drizzle with 1 tablespoon of the olive oil, and place flesh-side down on the prepared baking sheet. Roast until browned and tender, about 35 minutes.

Meanwhile, in a heavy-bottomed saucepan, melt the coconut oil over medium heat. Add the onion and a pinch of salt, stir, then reduce the heat to medium-low. Cover the pot and cook, stirring occasionally, for about 20 minutes, or until the onion is very soft and sweet.

Add the garlic, ginger, cumin, coriander, and garam masala, increase the heat to medium-high, and cook, stirring, for 1 minute. When the spices are fragrant but not burnt, add the stock and a big pinch of salt. Partially cover the pot and let the soup simmer gently while the squash roasts.

Let the squash cool slightly, then scrape the flesh into a bowl (discard the skin); you should have about 2 cups cooked squash. Add the squash to the pot with the stock and bring the soup to a boil. Reduce the heat to maintain a simmer, partially cover the pot, and cook for 10 minutes.

Carefully transfer the soup to a blender and blend until smooth (work in batches, if necessary, and be careful when blending hot liquids). Alternatively, blend the soup directly in the pot with an immersion blender. Taste for seasoning, ladle or pour into bowls, and enjoy!

Beet Gazpacho

QUICK / VEGAN

Serves 2

Cold soup can sometimes feel a little less than satisfying, but this beet gazpacho is somehow rich and even feels a little indulgent. Topped with diced cucumber and avocado, it's a perfect hot-day lunch that even the toughest gazpacho naysayer can get behind.

FOR THE GAZPACHO:

2 cups chopped Roasted Beets (page 198)

¼ red onion, chopped (about ⅓ cup)

2 garlic cloves

2 Persian cucumbers, peeled and seeded (about 1 cup)

½ cup water

Juice of 1 lemon

½ teaspoon kosher salt

1 teaspoon apple cider vinegar

TO GARNISH:

Finely diced cucumber

Avocado

Fresh cilantro leaves

Combine all the gazpacho ingredients in a high-speed blender and blend until smooth. Pour into small bowls and garnish with cucumber, avocado, and cilantro.

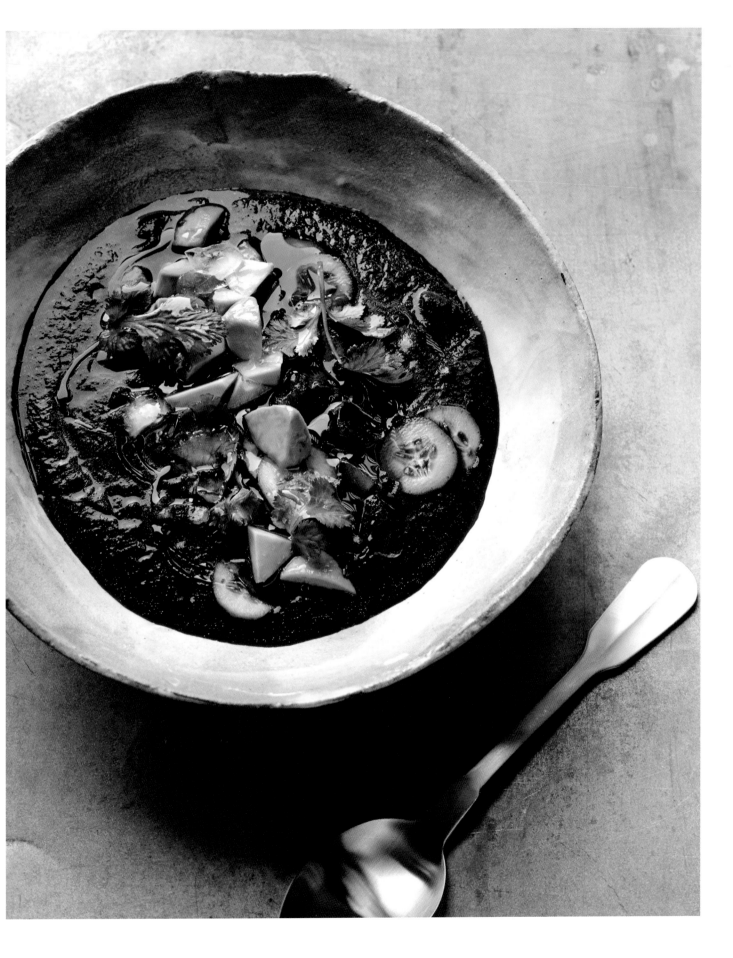

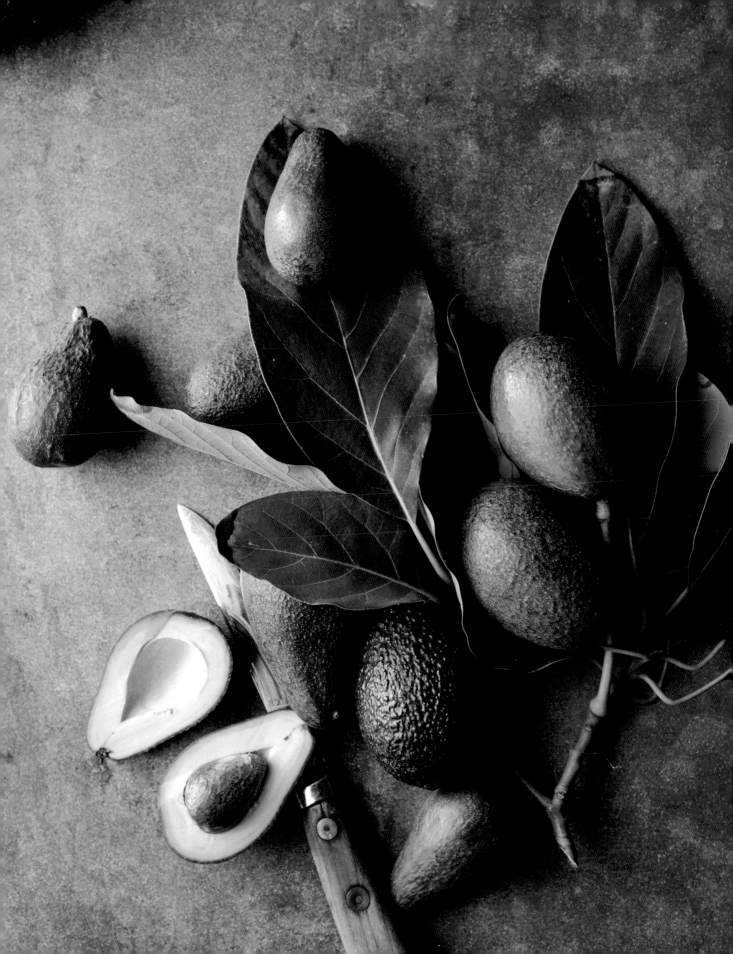

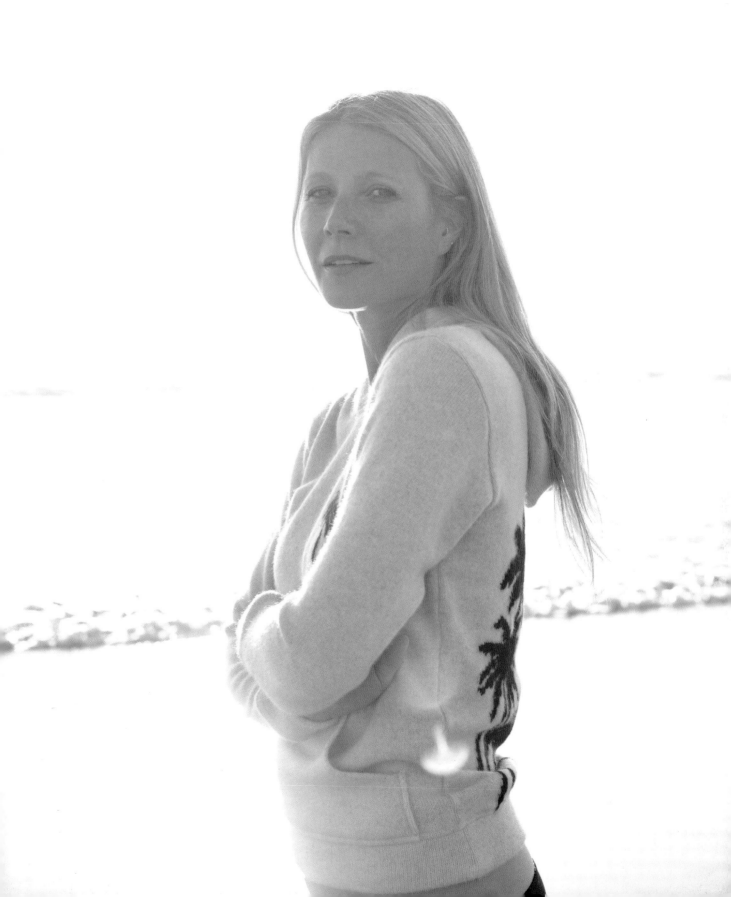

Cucumber & Avocado Gazpacho

QUICK / VEGAN

Serves 2

This easy, bright cucumber gazpacho makes a lovely light lunch or first course for a summer dinner party.

FOR THE GAZPACHO:

1 large seedless English cucumber, peeled

¼ avocado

1 large scallion, roughly chopped

1 garlic clove, grated

¼ cup olive oil

¼ cup plus 2 tablespoons water

1 teaspoon kosher salt, plus more as needed

2 tablespoons apple cider vinegar

TO GARNISH:

Finely chopped fresh mint leaves

Apple cider vinegar

Flaky sea salt

1 small shallot, finely diced

Olive oil

Cracked black pepper

To make the gazpacho, cut a 2-inch piece off the end of the cucumber and set it aside for garnish. Roughly chop the remaining cucumber and transfer it to a high-speed blender.

Add the avocado, scallion, garlic, olive oil, water, kosher salt, and vinegar and blend until smooth. Chill in the fridge for at least 1 hour.

For the garnish, finely dice the reserved piece of cucumber and toss in a small bowl with the mint leaves, apple cider vinegar, a pinch of flaky salt, and minced shallot.

Remove the gazpacho from the fridge, taste, and season with kosher salt. Divide between two bowls and spoon over the chopped cucumber relish. Drizzle each bowl with olive oil and finish with cracked pepper.

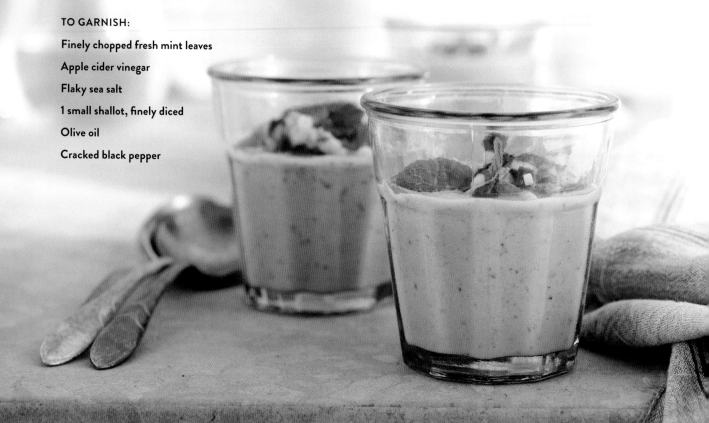

Coconut Chicken Soup

Serves 2

I'm a sucker for Thai food and especially love *tom kha gai*—a chicken soup made with lemongrass, galangal, coconut milk, and fish sauce, one of my favorite ingredients. This is my cleaned-up version, which, while not exactly authentic, is still pretty damn delicious.

1 tablespoon coconut oil

2 tablespoons finely minced fresh ginger

1 tablespoon finely minced garlic

3 tablespoons chopped fresh cilantro (leaves and stems)

2 cups Chicken Stock (page 193)

1 (16-ounce) can full-fat coconut milk

1 lemongrass stalk, smashed

1 boneless, skinless chicken breast, cut into thin strips

2 tablespoons coconut aminos

1½ tablespoons fish sauce

2 heads of baby bok choy, roughly chopped

½ cup snap peas

1 small zucchini, spiralized

Juice of 1 lime

In a 4-quart Dutch oven, melt the coconut oil over medium heat. Add the ginger, garlic, and cilantro and cook, stirring, for 30 seconds, or until fragrant but not browned.

Add the stock, coconut milk, and lemongrass and bring to a simmer. Add the chicken, coconut aminos, and fish sauce and cook for 5 to 7 minutes, until the chicken is just cooked through. Stir in the bok choy, snap peas, and zucchini noodles.

Divide the soup between two bowls. Squeeze over fresh lime juice just before serving.

Chicken Meatball Pho

Serves 2

I crave this warming ginger-infused soup whenever I'm feeling a little under the weather. Make a double batch of both the broth and the meatballs and freeze half, so you can whip this up at a moment's notice.

FOR THE BROTH:

4 cups Chicken Stock (page 193)

1 (2-inch) piece fresh ginger, sliced

3 garlic cloves, smashed

2 star anise pods

½ cinnamon stick

12 cilantro sprigs

Kosher salt (optional)

FOR THE MEATBALLS:

½ pound ground dark meat chicken

2 tablespoons finely chopped cilantro

2 tablespoons finely chopped basil

2 scallions, minced

Grated zest of ½ lime

¼ teaspoon kosher salt

TO FINISH:

1 small zucchini, spiralized

¼ cup bean sprouts

1 scallion, thinly sliced

Fresh cilantro leaves

Torn fresh basil leaves

Lime wedges

To make the broth, combine all the broth ingredients in a 4-quart Dutch oven and bring to a boil. Reduce the heat to medium-low, cover, and simmer gently for 15 minutes to infuse the flavors.

While the broth simmers, make the meatballs. Combine all the meatball ingredients in a medium bowl and roll into 1-inch meatballs.

Fish the aromatics out of the broth and discard them. Taste the broth and season with salt, if needed. Add the meatballs to the broth, cover the pot with the lid ajar, and gently simmer the meatballs for about 10 minutes.

Divide the zucchini between two bowls and top with the broth and meatballs. Garnish with the bean sprouts, scallions, cilantro, and basil and serve with lime wedges for squeezing.

Chicken & Leek Soup

Serves 2

This is a staple in the UK (where it's known as cock-a-leekie soup)—it's the kind of recipe everyone's mother or grandmother has. While the original is thickened with barley, my version is thick and rich from all the leeks. When cooked down and caramelized, they almost act as noodles.

2 tablespoons olive oil

2 or 3 leeks, washed well and thinly sliced (about 4 cups)

1 teaspoon kosher salt

2 rosemary sprigs

1 boneless, skinless chicken breast

4 cups Chicken Stock (page 193)

Flaky sea salt and cracked black pepper

In a medium Dutch oven, heat the olive oil over medium heat. Add the leeks and kosher salt, stir well, and simmer for 5 to 8 minutes, until the leeks have wilted and begun to caramelize.

Add the rosemary, chicken, and stock. Cover and cook for 20 to 25 minutes, until the chicken is opaque and cooked through.

Remove the chicken and set aside to cool. Increase the heat to medium-high and bring the soup to a low boil. Cook for about 10 minutes, until the soup has thickened.

When the chicken is cool enough to handle, shred it.

Remove and discard the rosemary sprigs and return the shredded chicken to the pot. Finish the soup with flaky salt and cracked pepper and serve.

Peruvian Chicken Cauli Rice Soup

Serves 2

A friend of mine told me about this soup she'd had at a Peruvian restaurant called *aguadito de pollo* that was a vibrant green color from all the cilantro in it. As a lover of cilantro for its unmistakable flavor, I had to try to make my own version of the soup. After tinkering a bit and swapping out the rice for cauliflower rice, I landed on a soup that was equal parts light and satiating. Cilantro is said to have chelating properties—meaning it may help the body get rid of heavy metals (see page 227)—and is generally thought of as a cleansing herb in the Ayurvedic tradition (see page 252). This is the kind of cleanse-friendly food I'd eat whenever.

1 medium white onion, chopped

1 bunch of cilantro, roughly chopped

½ jalapeño (optional)

Juice of 3 limes

¼ cup water, plus more if needed

4 cups Chicken Stock (page 193)

1 boneless, skinless chicken breast

1 teaspoon kosher salt

½ head of cauliflower, riced (1 to 1½ cups)

½ cup frozen peas

Lime wedges, for serving

Combine the onion, cilantro, jalapeño (if using), lime juice, and water in a high-speed blender and blend until smooth, adding a little extra water if needed to loosen the mixture. Set aside.

In a medium soup pot, bring the stock to a simmer over medium-low heat. Add the chicken and salt and cook until the chicken is opaque and fully cooked through, about 20 minutes. Remove the chicken and let cool.

Meanwhile, add the cauliflower rice and peas to the broth and simmer for 10 to 15 minutes, until the cauliflower rice is tender but not mushy.

When the chicken is cool enough to handle, shred the meat.

To serve, increase the heat to medium, return the shredded chicken to the pot, and add the onion-cilantro puree. Stir to combine and cook for 5 minutes before serving.

Divide into bowls and garnish with lime.

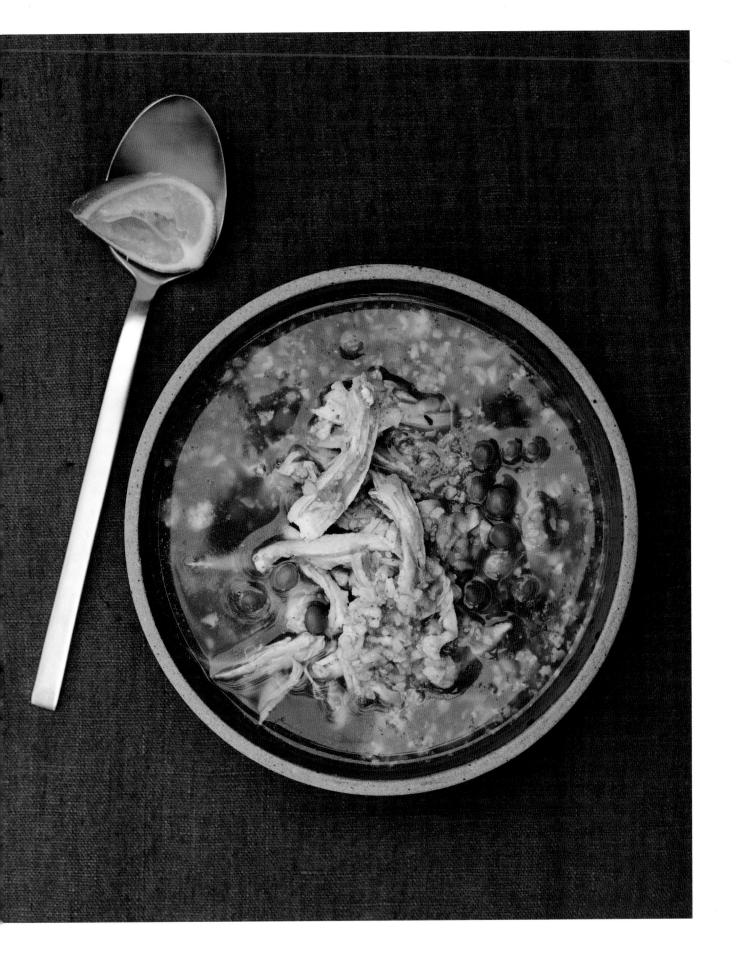

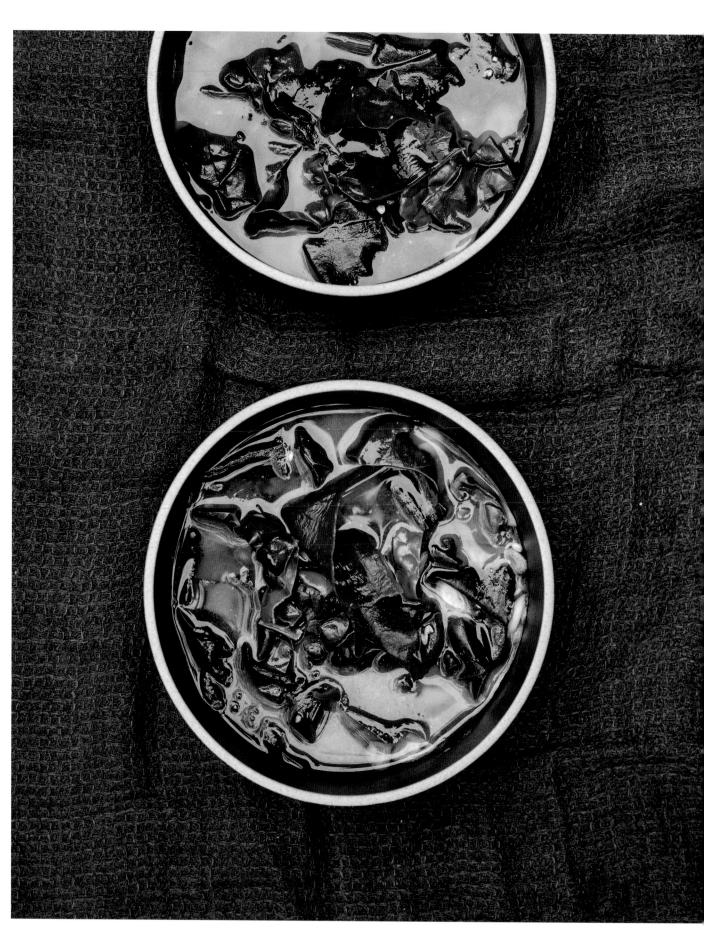

Miso Soup

QUICK / VEGAN

Serves 2

Probiotic-rich, gut-healing miso—combined with the kind of greens that many functional doctors have told me to add to my diet over the years—is another soup I turn to when something's ailing me. If you haven't tried cooking with wakame yet, it's the seaweed you normally find in miso soup, and it's a source of minerals like iron. You can find it in health food stores, or often in the Asian foods aisle of the grocery store (and, of course, you can always find it online).

4 cups cool water

2 tablespoons dried instant wakame

3 to 4 tablespoons chickpea miso paste

½ cup hot water

½ cup chopped Swiss chard

½ cup thinly sliced scallions

Kosher salt (optional)

In a medium saucepan, bring the water to a boil. Add wakame, reduce the heat to medium and simmer for 4 to 6 minutes.

Place 3 tablespoons of the miso in a small bowl, add the hot water, and whisk until the miso is smooth. Stir the miso mixture into the pot with the wakame.

Add the chard and scallions to the pot and cook over medium-high heat for 5 minutes. Taste and add more miso or season with salt, if desired.

Serve warm.

Brown Rice, Turmeric & Spinach Porridge

Serves 2

This spinach and brown rice porridge—a flavor and texture mash-up of Chinese congee and Indian dal—is endlessly comforting. I like it garnished with a large spoonful of cilantro salsa verde, but roughly chopped cilantro and a spoonful of unsweetened coconut yogurt also work well.

2 tablespoons coconut oil

1 small bunch of scallions, thinly sliced

1 (2-inch) piece fresh ginger, peeled and very finely minced or grated

4 large garlic cloves, very finely minced or grated

1 teaspoon ground turmeric

½ cup short-grain brown rice

4 cups Chicken Stock or Vegetable Stock (pages 193 and 192)

1 cup water

Kosher salt and freshly ground black pepper

5 ounces baby spinach leaves, roughly chopped

Cilantro Salsa Verde (page 185; optional)

Lime wedges, for serving

In a small Dutch oven, melt the coconut oil over medium heat.

Add the scallions, ginger, and garlic and cook, stirring, for 2 minutes, or until fragrant but not browned.

Add the turmeric and brown rice and stir to coat the rice in the aromatics.

Pour in the stock and water and season generously with salt and pepper. Bring the mixture to a boil, then cover and reduce the heat to maintain a low simmer. Cook for 1 hour, stirring every 10 minutes or so to make sure the rice isn't sticking.

Stir in the baby spinach, cover, and cook for 2 minutes more. Season with salt and pepper.

Ladle into bowls and dollop each serving with a spoonful of salsa verde, if desired. Serve with lime wedges for squeezing.

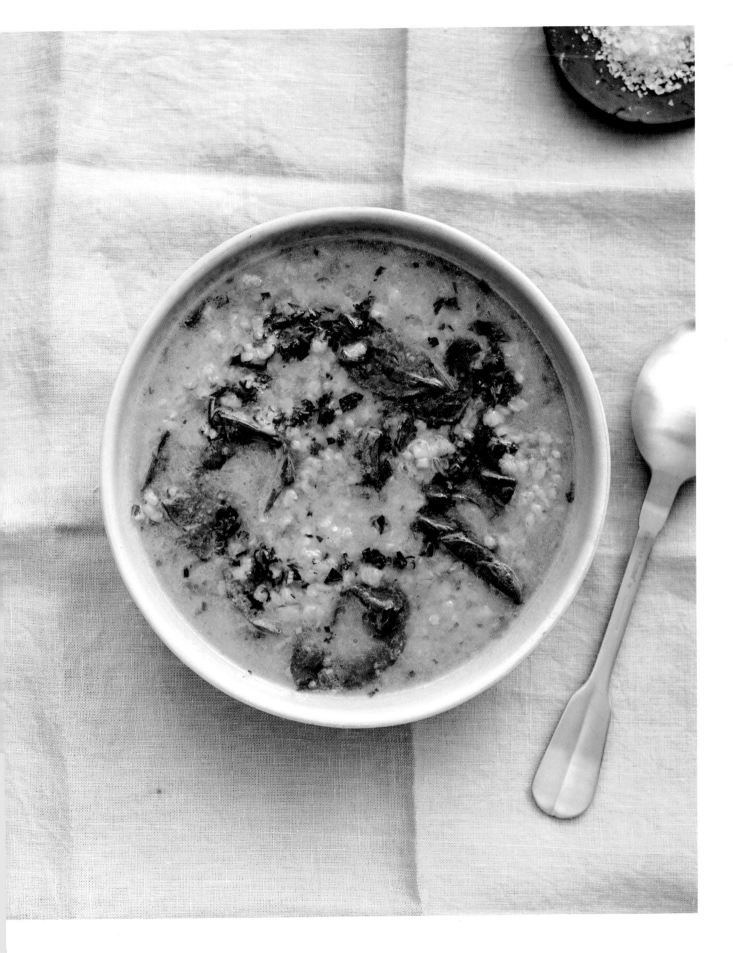

Broccoli-Parsnip Soup

VEGAN

Serves 2

Cleaning up broccoli soup can feel like a losing game (Uh, no cheese? No cream? Why bother?), but the natural sweetness and creaminess of parsnips saves the day. Even my kids love it. This recipe freezes well, so feel free to double up for a rainy day.

3 tablespoons olive oil

½ yellow onion, diced

½ teaspoon kosher salt

1 medium parsnip, peeled and diced

2 cups water

2 cups Vegetable Stock (page 192)

10 ounces broccoli, cut into florets

Flaky sea salt and cracked black pepper

In a heavy-bottomed pot, heat the olive oil over medium heat. Add the onion and cook for 5 to 7 minutes, until softened and beginning to caramelize. Add the kosher salt, parsnip, water, and stock. Cover, increase the heat to medium-high, and cook for about 20 minutes, or until the parsnips are soft. Add the broccoli, cover, and cook for about 10 minutes, or until the broccoli is fork-tender. Remove from the heat.

Working in batches as needed, carefully transfer the soup to a high-speed blender and blend until smooth (be careful when blending hot liquids). Alternatively, blend the soup directly in the pot with an immersion blender.

Finish with flaky salt and cracked pepper and serve.

Chickpea
& Escarole Soup

Serves 4

A cross between a soup and a stew, this interpretation of a classic Italian recipe gets real depth of flavor from sweet, sticky roasted garlic. If you can't find escarole, any sturdy green can stand in.

1 head of garlic, cloves separated and peeled

5 tablespoons olive oil

1 small or ½ large yellow onion, finely diced

1 carrot, diced

2 celery stalks, diced

1 teaspoon fennel seeds

¼ teaspoon chili flakes

6 cups Chicken Stock or Vegetable Stock (pages 193 and 192)

2 (14-ounce) cans chickpeas, drained and rinsed

Kosher salt

1 small bunch of escarole, leaves roughly torn and cleaned

Lemon zest, for serving

Parsley Salsa Verde (page 183), for serving

Flaky sea salt and cracked black pepper

Preheat the oven to 325°F.

Place the garlic cloves in a small ramekin and pour over 2 tablespoons of the olive oil. Cover with parchment paper and bake for 25 minutes.

Meanwhile, in a medium Dutch oven, heat the remaining 3 tablespoons of olive oil over medium heat. Add the onion, carrot, celery, fennel seeds, and chili flakes and cook for 10 minutes, or until the vegetables are translucent and just starting to brown.

Add the stock and half the chickpeas, and season with kosher salt. Bring the soup to a boil, then reduce the heat to maintain a simmer, cover the pot with the lid ajar, and cook for 20 minutes.

Remove the garlic from the oven. Using a fork, lift out all the roasted cloves and add them to the soup, reserving the infused oil.

Remove the soup from the heat. Blend the soup directly in the pot with an immersion blender until smooth. Stir in the remaining chickpeas and the escarole and cook over medium-high heat for 10 minutes more.

Ladle into bowls. Serve topped with a drizzle of the reserved garlic oil, some lemon zest, a spoonful of salsa verde, and flaky salt and cracked black pepper.

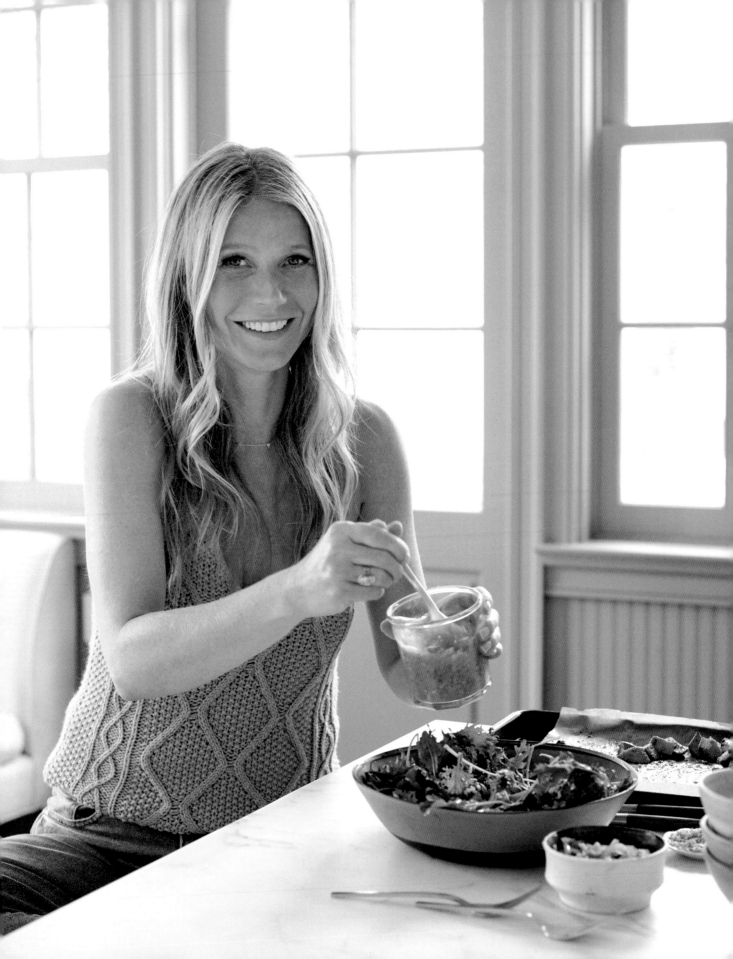

SALADS, BOWLS & ROLLS

Chopped salads, summer rolls, nori wraps, and Buddha bowls: I eat some sort of crunchy, veggie-packed salad, bowl, or roll for lunch almost every single day. It's not so much about eating clean, it's just that few dishes can continually satisfy me as much come one p.m. They're healthy and endlessly versatile—you can usually sub in whatever mix of veggies, proteins, and sauces you have on hand. The real selling point, though, might be their portability. Lunch is the worst meal to leave up to chance, in my experience, because I usually end up disappointed after the what-to-order scramble is over. With a little prep and some good nontoxic storage containers (Onyx makes the best stainless steel ones), I can eat nourishing, fresh, and totally satisfying lunches whether I'm at home, in the office, on set, or en route to a meeting. So for anyone who is always on the go, which seems to be just about everyone these days, these make-ahead, packable, clean-eating dream recipes are for you.

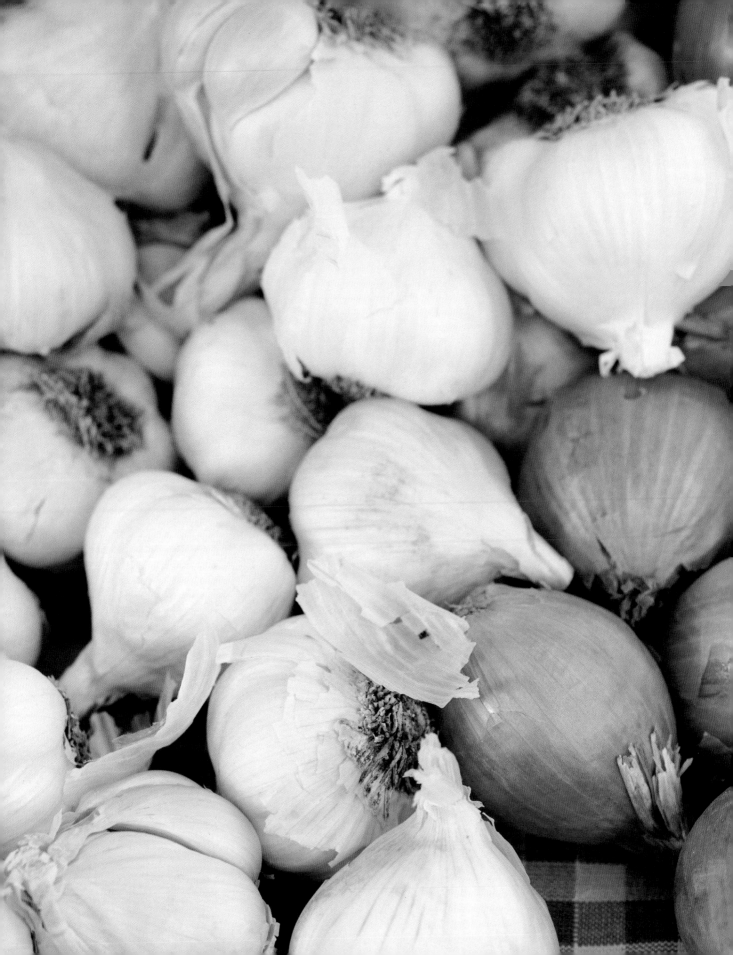

Grilled Chicken Salad with Miso Dressing

<u>PACKABLE</u>

Serves 2

A crunchy, gingery salad with grilled chicken has been my jam for longer than I can remember. This one feels super hydrating with the snap peas and jicama, and that grilled chicken adds some heft to help you power through the four o'clock snack slump.

FOR THE CHICKEN:

1 garlic clove, peeled and grated

1 (1-inch) piece fresh ginger

½ teaspoon toasted sesame oil

2 tablespoons coconut aminos

¼ teaspoon kosher salt

1 chicken breast cutlet

Sunflower seed oil

FOR THE SALAD:

1 cup shredded romaine

½ cup chopped snap peas

¼ cup julienned jicama

¼ cup bean sprouts

4 scallions, thinly sliced

Miso-Ginger Dressing (page 188)

½ teaspoon sesame seeds, to garnish

To make the chicken, in a medium bowl, whisk together the garlic, ginger, sesame oil, coconut aminos, and salt. Add the chicken and marinate at room temperature for 15 to 20 minutes.

Heat a grill pan over medium-high heat. Brush the pan with a little sunflower seed oil, then add the chicken and cook for 3 to 5 minutes on each side, depending on the thickness. When done, set aside to rest for a few minutes, then slice into ½-inch-thick strips.

To make the salad, in a serving bowl, toss together all the salad ingredients.

Drizzle the salad with the dressing and top with the sliced grilled chicken and sesame seeds.

Carrot & Beet Slaw

PACKABLE / QUICK / VEGAN

Serves 4

If you get tired of green salads, try rotating this into the mix. Shredded raw beets, carrots, herbs, and a little bit of apple cider vinegar make a bright and satisfying salad that would go with just about anything. In an ideal world, I love it to balance the richness of a burger. Seriously, serve this at a BBQ and everyone will be too busy eating it to even realize how clean it is.

2 cups grated carrots

1½ cups grated beets

4 scallions, thinly sliced

½ teaspoon kosher salt

¼ cup plus 1 tablespoon apple cider vinegar

Combine all the ingredients in a medium bowl. Cover and let sit for 5 to 10 minutes before serving.

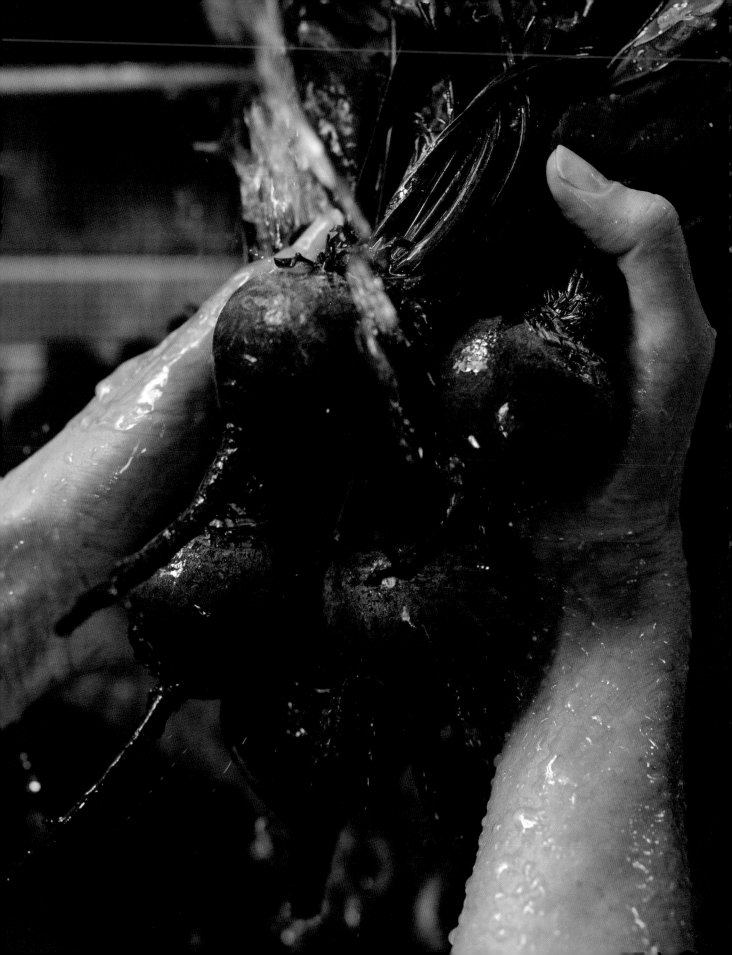

Italian Chicken Salad with Grilled Asparagus

Serves 2

I love chicories like radicchio, frisée, and escarole, but I get that not everyone is into their bitter flavor. The trick here is balancing those flavors with peppery arugula, sweet fennel, and super-savory grilled chicken and asparagus. This way you can enjoy the digestive benefits of these greens without the intense bitterness.

Zest of 1 lemon

2 garlic cloves, grated

½ teaspoon fresh thyme leaves

¼ cup extra virgin olive oil, plus more as needed

½ teaspoon kosher salt

¼ teaspoon chili flakes (optional)

1 chicken breast cutlet

½ bunch of asparagus

½ cup arugula

½ cup chopped radicchio

½ cup thinly sliced fennel

½ lemon

Flaky sea salt and cracked black pepper

In a small bowl, whisk together the lemon zest, garlic, thyme, olive oil, kosher salt, and chili flakes (if using). Divide the marinade between two medium bowls. Toss the chicken breast with the marinade in one bowl and the asparagus in the other, and let them sit for at least 30 minutes.

Heat a grill pan over high heat. Add the chicken and asparagus and cook for 4 minutes on each side until the chicken is fully cooked and the asparagus is nicely charred.

Meanwhile, in a serving bowl, toss together the arugula, radicchio, and fennel.

Cut the chicken and asparagus into bite-sized pieces, then squeeze the lemon half over them. Add the chicken and asparagus to the bowl with the greens and toss, adding a little more lemon juice and olive oil as needed.

Finish with flaky salt and cracked pepper and serve.

Garden Salad with Aquafaba Ranch Dressing

PACKABLE / QUICK / VEGAN

Serves 2

Sometimes you just want a crunchy garden salad! It's easy, healthy, tasty, and—who am I kidding—really just a vehicle for that aquafaba ranch.

1 cup shredded romaine lettuce

1 chopped Persian cucumber

¼ cup grated carrot

¼ cup chopped snap peas

½ avocado, diced

½ cup canned chickpeas

Aquafaba Ranch Dressing (page 181)

Combine all the ingredients except the dressing in a medium bowl. Add a few tablespoons of the dressing and toss. Divide the salad between two smaller bowls and serve.

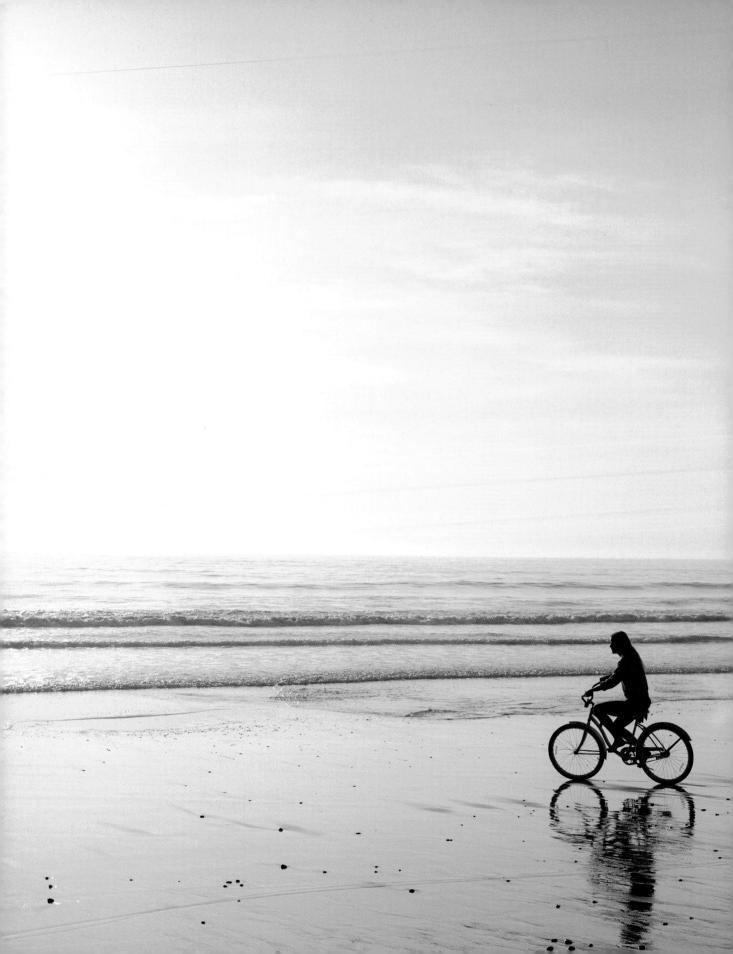

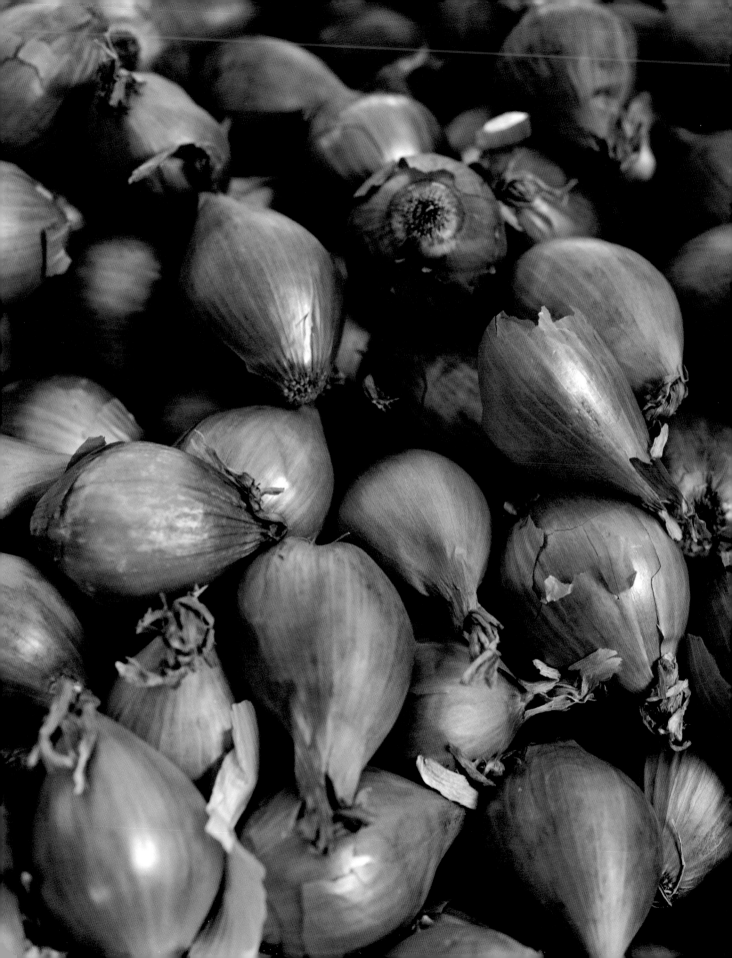

Greek Salad

PACKABLE / QUICK / VEGAN

Serves 2

From the protein-packed chickpeas to the crunch of the cucumbers, this bright green salad is a ten.

FOR THE DRESSING:

Juice of 1 lemon (about ¼ cup)

⅓ cup extra virgin olive oil

½ teaspoon kosher salt

1 tablespoon dried oregano

1 garlic clove

FOR THE SALAD:

1 head of romaine lettuce, chopped

1 Persian cucumber, diced

½ cup canned chickpeas

¼ cup Pickled Red Onions (page 206)

Kosher salt and freshly ground black pepper

To make the dressing, combine all the dressing ingredients in a high-speed blender and blend until well combined.

To make the salad, in a large salad bowl, combine all the ingredients for the salad and toss until well combined. Add the dressing and toss once more.

Finish with salt and pepper and serve.

Kale, Carrot & Avo Salad with Tahini Dressing

PACKABLE / QUICK / VEGAN

Serves 2

Adding grilled chicken to everything is an easy way to protein-pack a meal when you're eating clean, but it can get a little old. This salad is one of those meals I find satisfying without any animal protein, and it tends to please vegans and meat eaters alike. While I've dabbled in vegetarianism before, I don't see myself ever really going back. Still, I know that in essentially every hotbed of longevity in the world, people have followed a diet really limited in meat—so I try to take some cues from centenarians and keep meat from being too much a focus in my kitchen.

2 cups thinly sliced black kale leaves

1 cup grated carrots

Tahini Dressing (page 189)

1 avocado, thinly sliced

¼ cup sunflower seeds, toasted

In a serving bowl, toss the kale and carrots with a few tablespoons of the dressing, then top with the avocado and sunflower seeds and serve.

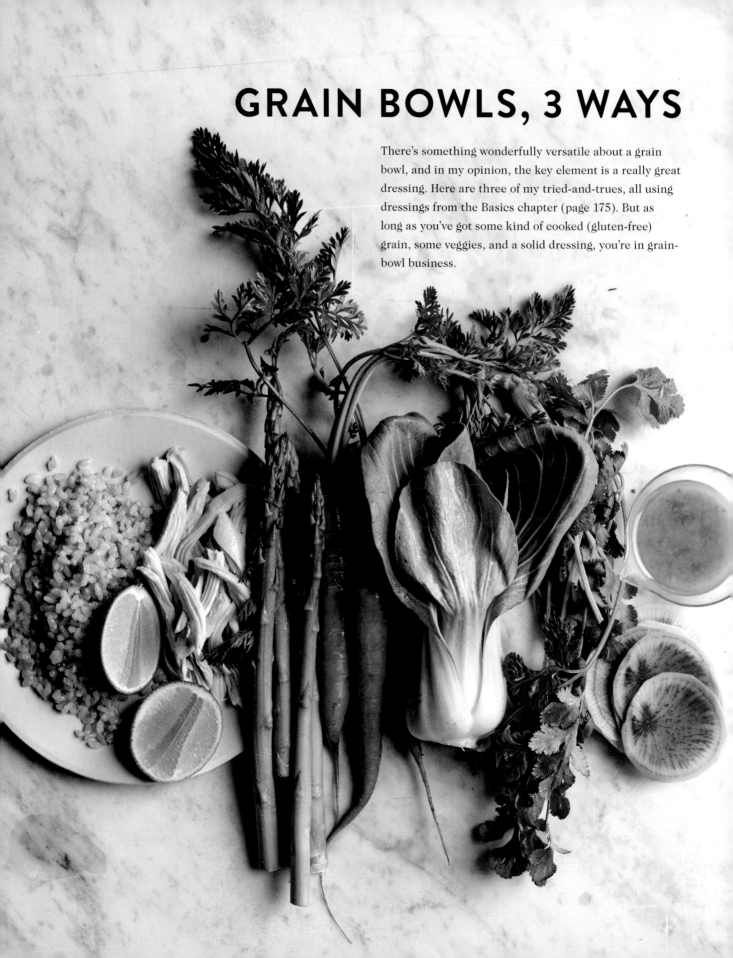

GRAIN BOWLS, 3 WAYS

There's something wonderfully versatile about a grain bowl, and in my opinion, the key element is a really great dressing. Here are three of my tried-and-trues, all using dressings from the Basics chapter (page 175). But as long as you've got some kind of cooked (gluten-free) grain, some veggies, and a solid dressing, you're in grain-bowl business.

Brown Rice Grain Bowl with Kale, Broccoli & Sesame

PACKABLE / VEGAN

Serves 2

If you're packing this for lunch (for you or your kiddos), cook the broccoli and make the dipping sauce the night before so all you have to do in the morning is assemble the bowls. A cruciferous vegetable, broccoli is a prized ingredient in a lot of doctors' books. But I didn't know until getting into Dr. Amy Myers's protocols that, because of its sulfur- and nitrogen-containing compounds, broccoli can be used as a tool in healing from Candida (for more info, see the Candida Reset on page 237).

Kosher salt

1 cup broccoli florets

1 cup cooked brown rice

½ cup grated carrot

½ cup finely chopped kale leaves

2 tablespoons toasted sesame seeds

Coconut Aminos Sauce (page 186)

Bring a saucepan of salted water to a boil. Fill a medium bowl with ice and water. Add the broccoli to the boiling water and cook for about 3 minutes, or until just tender. Drain the broccoli and shock it in the ice water to stop the cooking. Drain again.

To assemble, divide the brown rice between two bowls, then top each with half the broccoli, carrot, and kale. Sprinkle with the sesame seeds and drizzle with dipping sauce right before eating.

Crunchy Spring Veggie Grain Bowl

PACKABLE / QUICK

Serves 2

Spring in a bowl, this crunchy-salad-meets-grain-bowl is all I want to eat for lunch when it turns warm outside.

1 cup cooked quinoa or brown rice

3 asparagus spears, shaved

½ cup grated carrot

½ small watermelon radish, thinly sliced with a mandoline

⅔ cup shredded Poached Chicken (page 196; optional)

⅔ cup thinly sliced bok choy

¼ cup chopped fresh cilantro leaves

Miso-Ginger Dressing (page 188)

About 1 tablespoon coconut aminos

About 1 teaspoon toasted sesame oil

Divide the quinoa between two bowls. Top each with half the asparagus, carrot, radish, chicken, and bok choy. Garnish with the cilantro and pour over the miso dressing. Drizzle with the coconut aminos and sesame oil and serve.

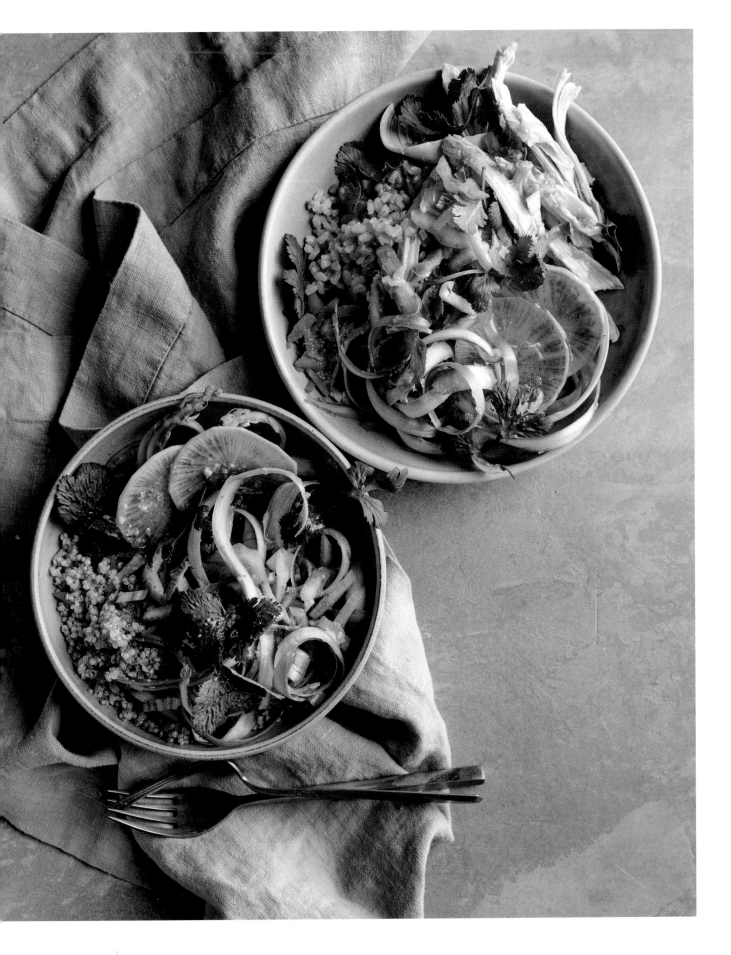

Quinoa, Sweet Potato & Tahini Grain Bowl

PACKABLE / VEGAN

Serves 2

The flavor combination of sweet potato and tahini is made even better here by the addition of earthy beets, spicy arugula, and creamy avocado. Yum.

1 small sweet potato, peeled and cut into 1-inch pieces

1 tablespoon olive oil

Kosher salt and freshly ground black pepper

1 cup cooked quinoa

⅔ cup cubed Roasted Beets (page 198)

⅔ cup baby arugula

½ avocado, diced

¼ cup sunflower seeds, toasted

Tahini Dressing (page 189)

Preheat the oven to 400°F. Line a baking sheet with parchment paper.

In a medium bowl, toss the sweet potato with the olive oil, season with salt and pepper, and place on the prepared baking sheet. Roast for 20 minutes, or until tender and lightly browned. Remove from the oven and let cool.

Divide the cooked quinoa between two bowls. Top each with half the sweet potato, beets, arugula, and avocado. Sprinkle with the sunflower seeds and pour over tahini dressing.

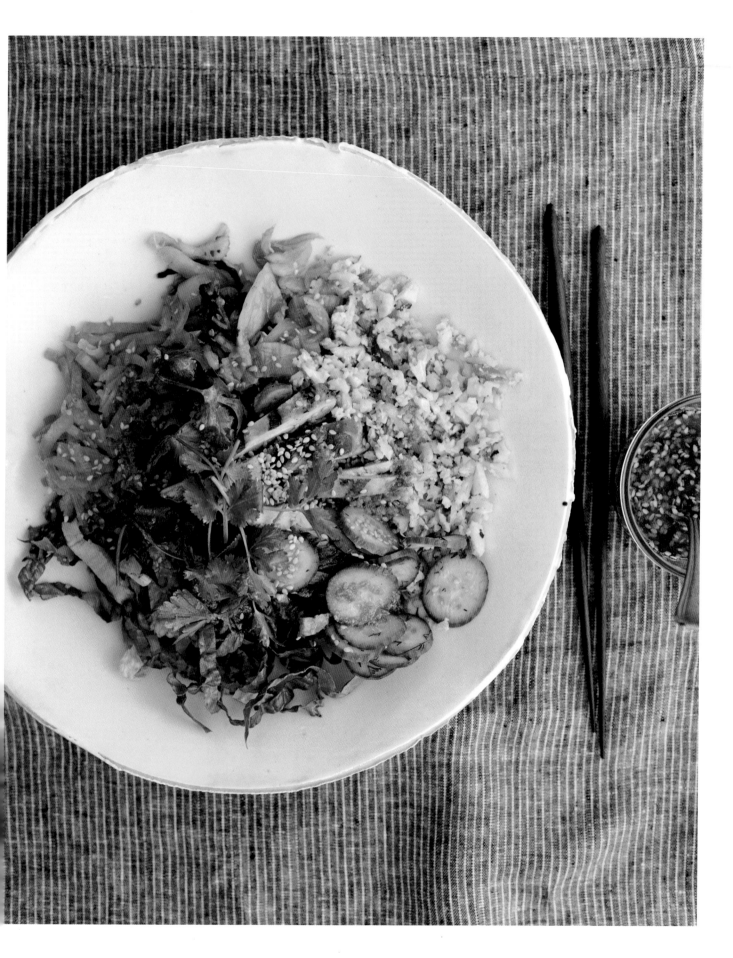

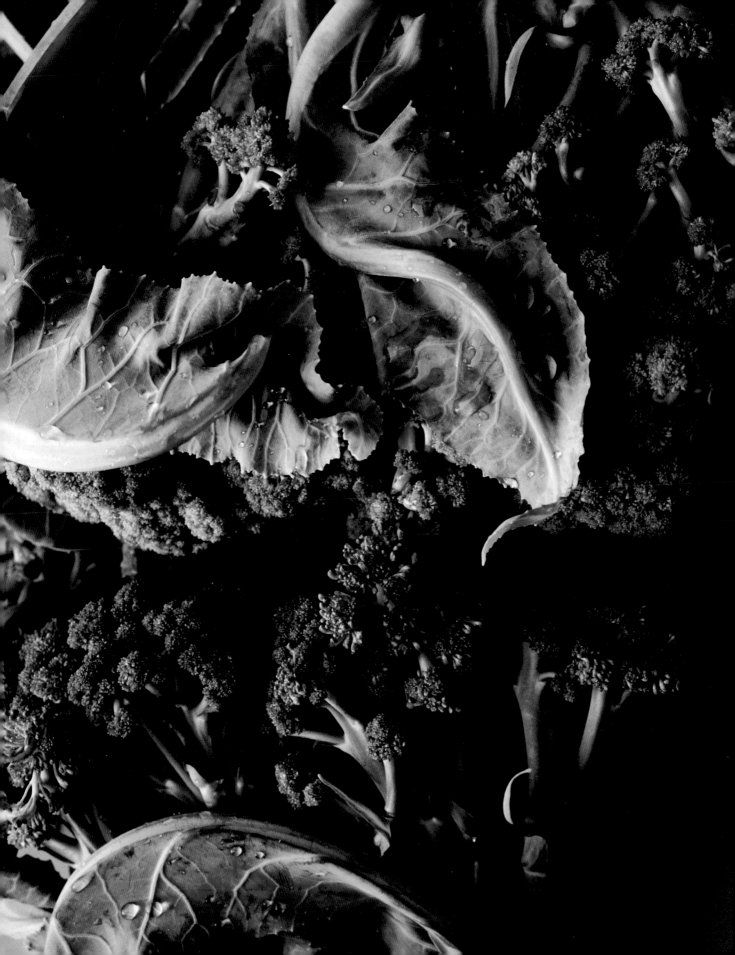

CAULIFLOWER BOWLS, 3 WAYS

If you're not doing grains, cauliflower rice is a major lifesaver. One of my favorite nutritionists, Shira Lenchewski, MS, RD, often recommends it as a healthy dinner option for the time-strapped. And these three cauli rice bowls are so good, you'll want to make them even if grains are part of your regular diet.

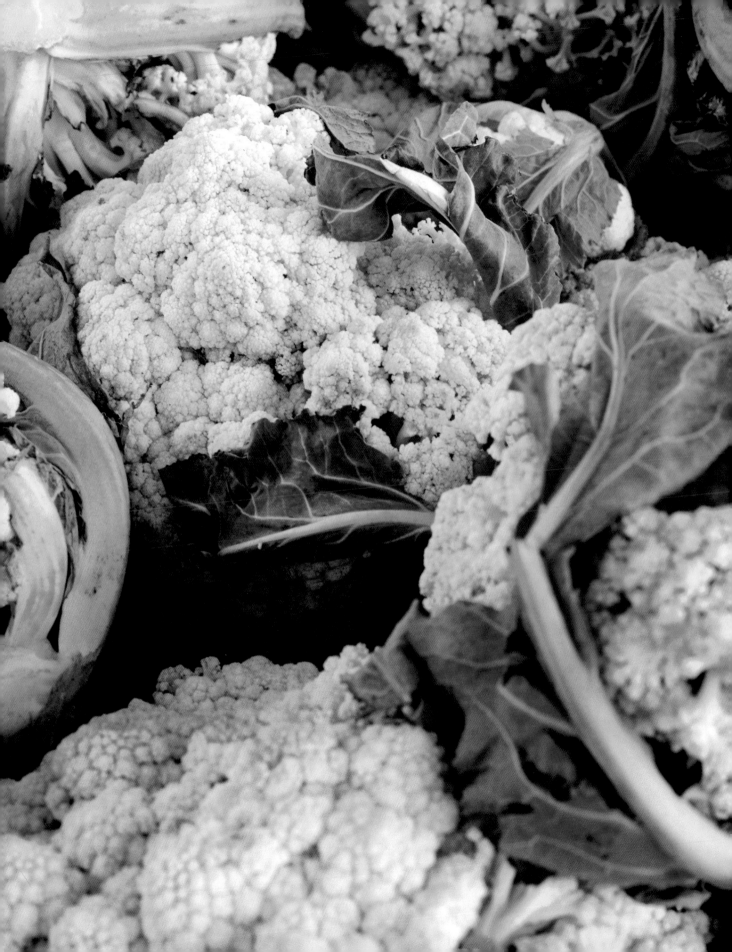

Teriyaki Bowl

PACKABLE

Serves 2

Whenever I make this, I double the marinated chicken. That way I can grill it up alongside veggies, serve it with a little cauli rice, drizzle it with some coconut aminos sauce, and dinner's served.

FOR THE TERIYAKI CHICKEN:

2 boneless, skinless chicken thighs (about ¾ pound)

1 small garlic clove, grated

1 teaspoon grated fresh ginger

¼ teaspoon kosher salt

2 tablespoons coconut aminos

Olive oil, for brushing the grill pan

FOR THE BOWL:

1 recipe Cauliflower Rice (page 211)

1 teaspoon toasted sesame oil

1 scallion, thinly sliced

¼ cup chopped romaine lettuce

¼ cup chopped kimchi

1 small carrot, grated

Pickled Cucumbers (page 209)

Fresh cilantro leaves

Toasted sesame seeds

Coconut Aminos Sauce (page 186)

To make the teriyaki chicken, combine the chicken thighs, garlic, ginger, salt, and coconut aminos in a small bowl and marinate at room temperature for 10 minutes.

Heat a grill pan over medium-high heat. Brush the pan with a little olive oil, add the chicken, and cook for 5 minutes per side, or until firm to the touch and cooked through. Transfer to a cutting board and let rest for at least 5 minutes.

Meanwhile, prepare the cauliflower rice, then stir in the toasted sesame oil and scallion. Divide the cauliflower rice between two bowls and top each with half the romaine, kimchi, carrot, and cucumber pickles.

Chop the grilled chicken and season with salt, if needed. Divide the chicken between the bowls and garnish each with cilantro leaves and sesame seeds. Pour a couple of tablespoons of the dipping sauce over each and serve with more sauce on the side.

Za'atar Chicken Bowl

Serves 2

This bowl combines some of my favorite things from Middle Eastern cuisine: grilled meat on a stick, tons of herbs and citrus, and a creamy, savory sauce to tie it all together. What more is there to say?

FOR THE CHICKEN:

1 boneless, skinless chicken breast, cut into 2-inch cubes

¼ red onion, cut into 2-inch cubes

1 tablespoon za'atar

1 teaspoon kosher salt

1 tablespoon olive oil, plus more as needed

FOR THE CAULIFLOWER RICE PILAF:

1 recipe Cauliflower Rice (page 211)

½ cup finely chopped black kale leaves (about 4 large leaves)

¼ cup minced fresh parsley

¼ cup minced fresh cilantro

¼ cup minced fresh chives

Zest of 1 lemon

Kosher salt

Tahini Dressing (page 189)

To make the chicken, in a medium bowl, combine the chicken, onion, za'atar, salt, and olive oil. Skewer the chicken and onion pieces, alternating them.

Heat a grill pan over high heat. Brush the pan with a little olive oil, add the skewers, and cook for about 5 minutes on each side, or until the chicken is cooked through and the onion is browned.

Meanwhile, make the cauliflower rice pilaf. Prepare the cauliflower rice, then add the kale and cook, stirring, for about 2 minutes, until slightly softened. Add the parsley, cilantro, chives, and lemon zest and cook for 1 minute more. Remove from the heat. Finish with a squeeze of lemon juice and some flaky salt.

Serve the skewers with the cauliflower rice pilaf and the dressing.

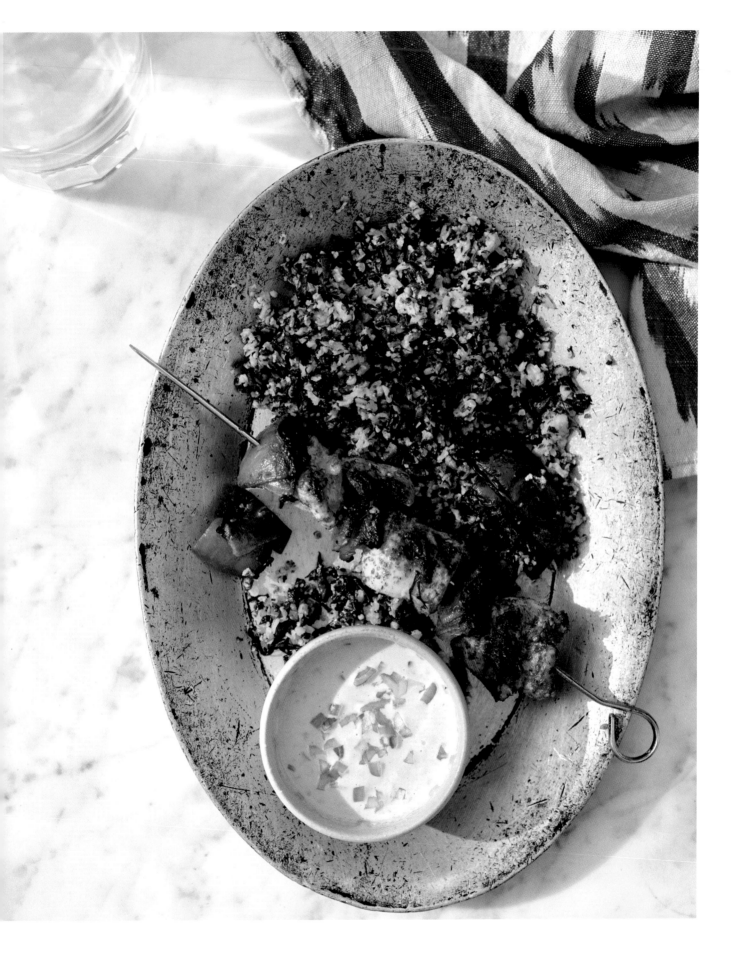

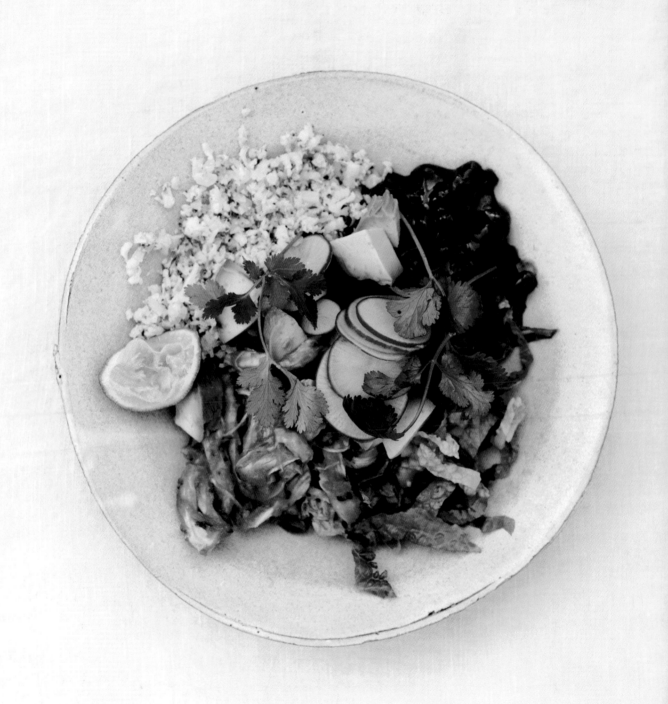

Tex-Mex Bowl

PACKABLE

Serves 2

Tostada salads are a popular lunch choice at goop, and while I can get down with a giant tortilla shell most days of the year, we wanted to create a version that didn't include corn, gluten, dairy, or nightshades. This is what I came up with—and I'm happy to say it's officially goop-approved.

1 recipe Cauliflower Rice (page 211)

Braised Mexican Nomato Chicken (page 140)

½ recipe Mexican Black Beans (page 201)

½ recipe Pickled Radishes (page 208)

¼ cup sliced romaine lettuce

½ avocado, chopped

Flaky sea salt

Cilantro leaves, to garnish

Lime wedges, for serving

Divide the cauliflower rice between two bowls. Top each with half the braised chicken, beans, pickled radishes, romaine, and avocado. Season with a little flaky salt and garnish with cilantro. Serve with lime wedges for squeezing.

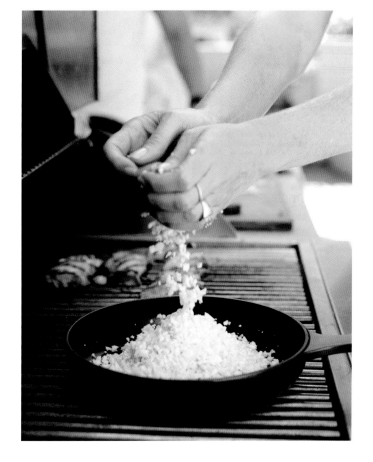

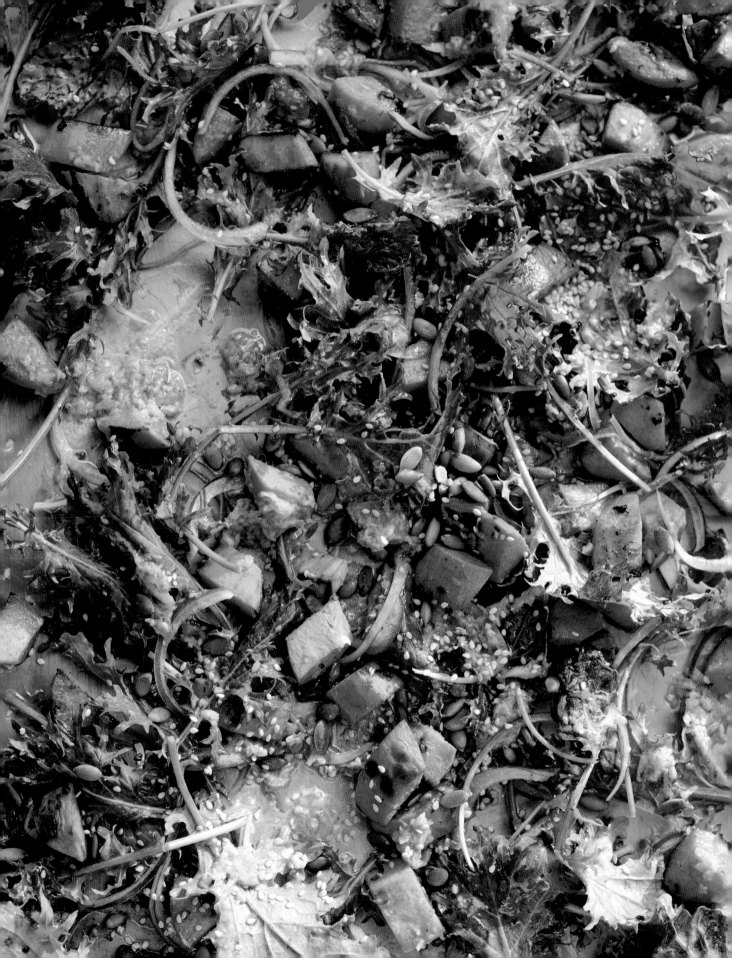

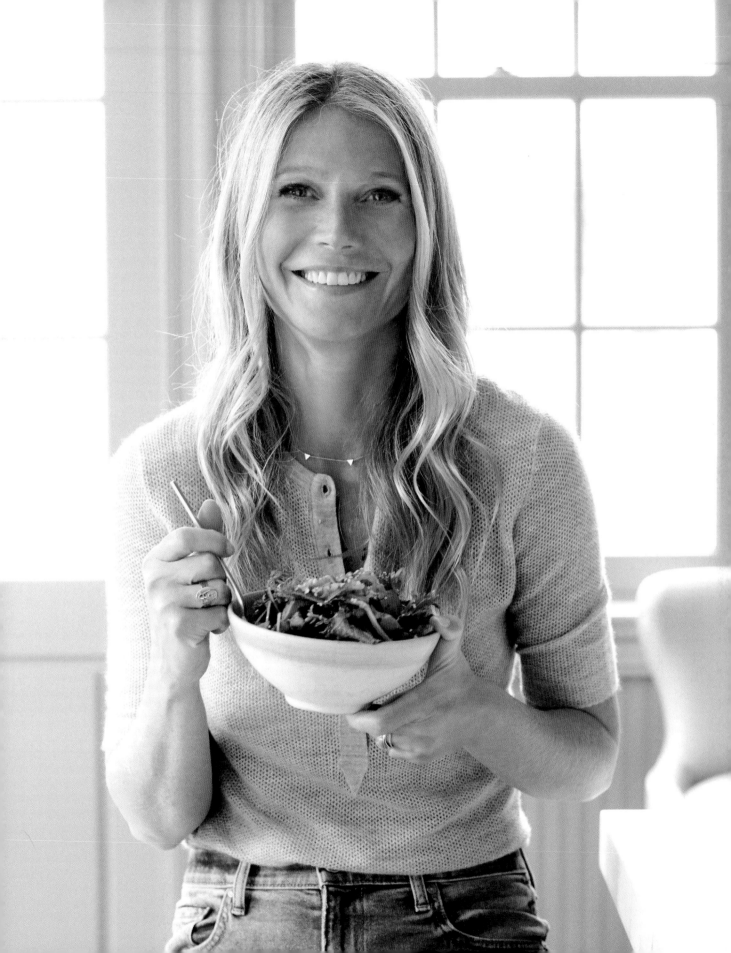

Kale & Sweet Potato Salad with Miso

PACKABLE / VEGAN

Serves 2

I could never get bored of this salad. It has some of my all-time favorite flavors (sweet potato, miso, ginger), and it's totally filling. Tossing the sweet potatoes with the dressing while they're still warm is key—it helps the potatoes absorb all that delicious citrusy-umami flavor.

1 tablespoon chickpea miso paste

2 tablespoons olive oil

1 sweet potato, cut into 1-inch cubes

⅛ medium red onion, thinly sliced

¼ teaspoon kosher salt

¼ teaspoon grated lime zest

2 cups baby kale

¼ cup picked fresh cilantro

¼ cup hulled pepitas (pumpkin seeds), toasted

Miso-Ginger Dressing (page 188)

1 teaspoon sesame seeds

Preheat the oven to 425°F. Line a baking sheet with parchment paper.

In a large bowl, whisk together the miso and olive oil. Toss the cubed sweet potatoes in the miso mixture until evenly coated. Spread the potatoes out on the prepared baking sheet and roast for 20 to 25 minutes, until soft and caramelized.

Meanwhile, in a small bowl, toss the onion slices with the salt and lime zest and let sit for about 10 minutes.

While the potatoes are still warm (not hot), transfer them to a serving bowl and toss with the kale, cilantro, pepitas, onion, and dressing. Finish with the sesame seeds.

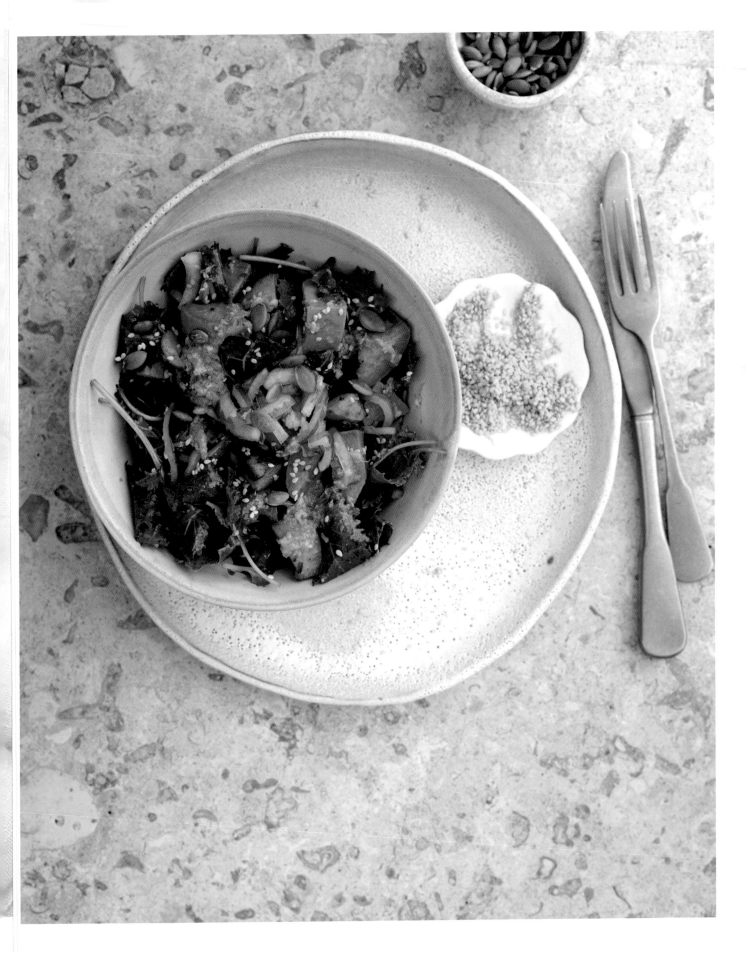

Tarragon Chicken Lettuce Cups

PACKABLE / QUICK

Serves 2

This is the most traditional of the three chicken salads, and that's precisely why it won me over. These flavors have been and always will be delicious together—plus, it's got the best textures: creamy, crunchy, and cool.

⅓ cup Aquafaba Mayo (page 178)

1 celery stalk, diced

1 small shallot, diced

1 tablespoon chopped fresh tarragon

¼ teaspoon kosher salt

1 poached chicken breast (page 196), shredded

Butter lettuce leaves, for serving

Cracked black pepper

Combine the mayo, celery, shallot, tarragon, and salt in a small bowl, then fold in the shredded chicken and mix thoroughly.

Arrange lettuce leaves on two plates. Spoon the mixture into the lettuce leaf cups and garnish with cracked pepper.

Chicken Larb Lettuce Cups

Serves 2

Another favorite dish of mine, this take on Thai chicken *larb*—flecked with fresh herbs and tossed in umami-rich fish sauce—is a staple in my house. Use ground dark meat chicken, which has way more flavor than white meat.

¾ pound ground dark meat chicken

½ bunch of scallions, thinly sliced

2 large garlic cloves, grated or finely minced

1 tablespoon grated fresh ginger

¾ teaspoon kosher salt

2 tablespoons olive oil

2 tablespoons coconut aminos

2 tablespoons fish sauce

6 large butter lettuce leaves

Thinly sliced red onion

1 tablespoon roughly chopped fresh mint leaves

1 tablespoon roughly chopped fresh cilantro leaves

1 tablespoon roughly chopped fresh Thai basil leaves

Lime wedges, for serving

In a medium bowl, combine the chicken, scallions, garlic, ginger, and salt.

In a large sauté pan, heat the olive oil over medium-high heat. Add the chicken and cook, stirring, until firm and no longer pink, about 8 minutes. Add the coconut aminos and fish sauce, stir to combine, and remove from the heat.

Divide the lettuce leaves between two plates. Fill the leaves with the chicken mixture and top each with some sliced red onion and the fresh herbs. Serve with lime wedges on the side for squeezing.

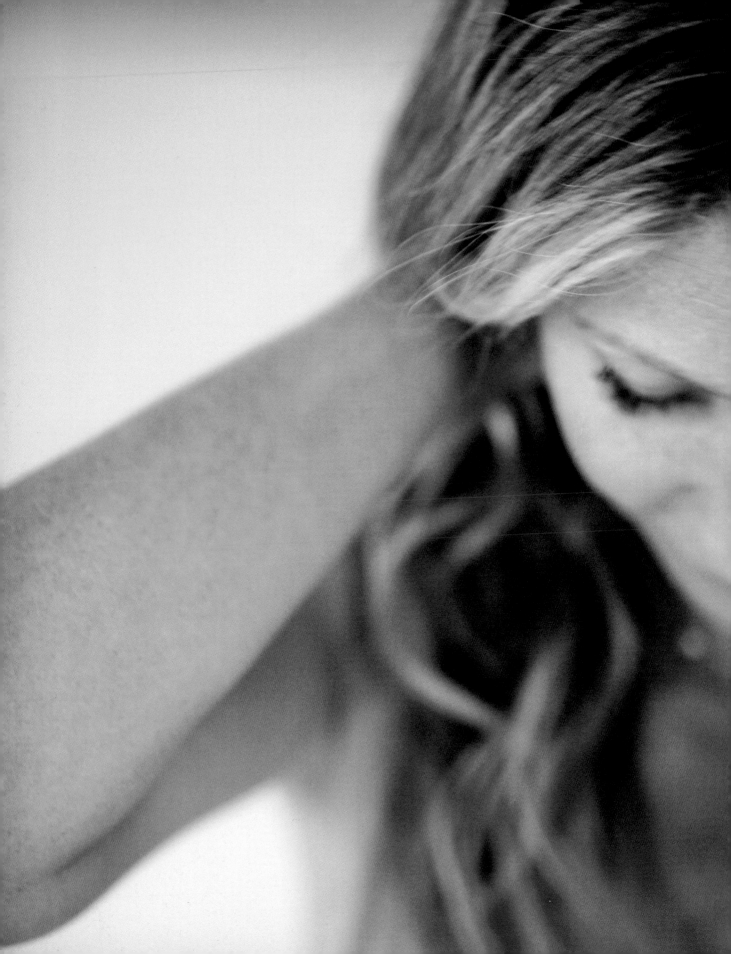

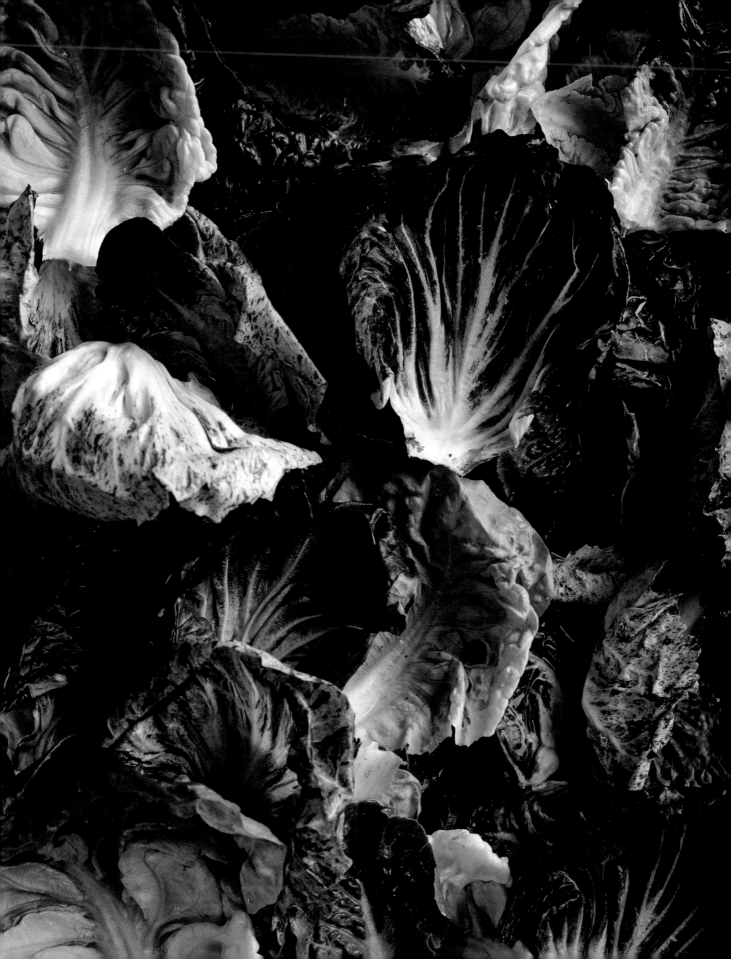

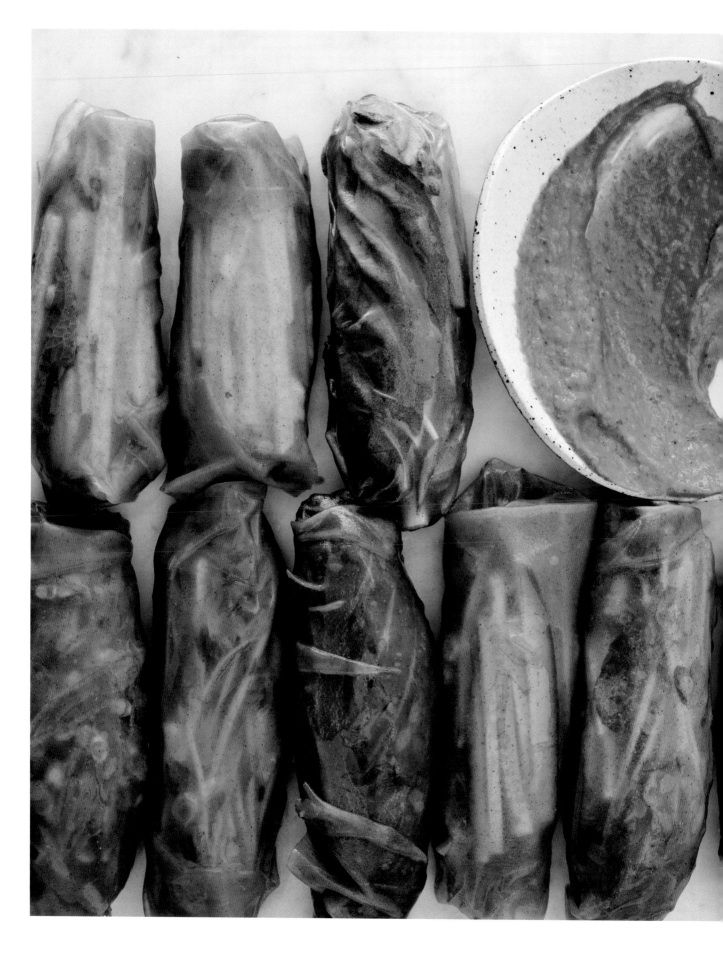

Crunchy Summer Rolls

PACKABLE / QUICK / VEGAN

Serves 2

I'm a huge fan of Vietnamese summer rolls, but most clean-eating protocols recommend steering clear of white rice. (Which I happen to really love. A little bowl of white rice with soy sauce is one of life's greatest pleasures. But I digress.) The game changer? Brown rice paper wrappers (typically found in the Asian foods aisle at the grocery store, or online). I stuff these with jicama, fresh herbs, and tons of green veggies, but fill them with any mix of herbs and veggies you like. Just don't forget the (addictive) creamy cashew dipping sauce!

FOR THE CASHEW SAUCE:

¼ cup unsweetened cashew butter

1 lime

1 teaspoon fish sauce

½ teaspoon grated fresh ginger

1 tablespoon water

2 garlic cloves

2 tablespoons coconut aminos

FOR THE SUMMER ROLLS:

4 to 6 brown rice paper wrappers

6 cilantro sprigs

2 Persian cucumbers, julienned

½ jicama, julienned

¾ cup thinly sliced snap peas

4 basil sprigs

4 mint sprigs

1½ cups mung bean sprouts

To make the cashew sauce, combine all the sauce ingredients in a high-speed blender and blend until smooth.

To assemble the rolls, fill a bowl large enough to hold the spring roll wrappers with warm water. Soak one wrapper for about 1 minute, or until just pliable, then lay it flat on a cutting board. Layer cilantro, cucumber, jicama, snap peas, basil, mint, and sprouts on the wrapper. Carefully roll up the wrapper, folding in the ends as you roll. Repeat with the remaining wrappers and filling ingredients.

Serve with the cashew sauce on the side. If not serving immediately, pack the rolls in an airtight container, layering them with damp paper towels to keep the rice paper moist.

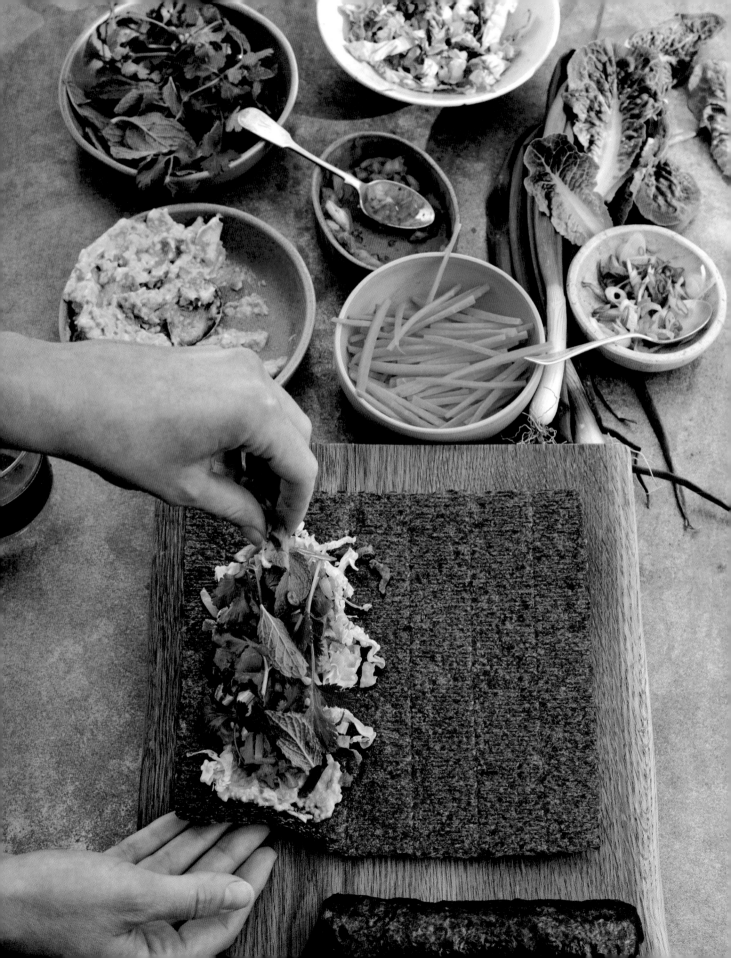

Nori Salad Roll

QUICK / VEGAN

Serves 2

I have these salad rolls, stuffed with good-for-your-gut kimchi, as a light lunch or afternoon snack. The nori can get a little soggy as it sits, so I try to eat the rolls soon after I assemble them. (This is not usually an issue for me, as they're totally delicious and I inhale them right away.)

1 avocado

Juice of 1 lime

4 sheets of nori

¾ cup finely chopped lettuce

1 medium carrot, julienned

½ cup chopped kimchi

4 mint sprigs

6 cilantro sprigs

Coconut Aminos Sauce (page 186), for serving

In a small bowl, mash together the avocado and lime juice.

Place the nori sheets flat on a cutting board. Top each nori sheet with a spoonful of the mashed avocado, spreading it evenly and leaving a ½-inch border. Top with the lettuce, carrots, kimchi, and herbs.

Working with one sheet at a time, lightly wet the top border of nori with water and, starting at the bottom, carefully roll up the nori around the filling as tightly as possible, using more water as necessary to hold the roll together. Repeat to roll up the remaining nori sheets.

Serve the rolls with dipping sauce.

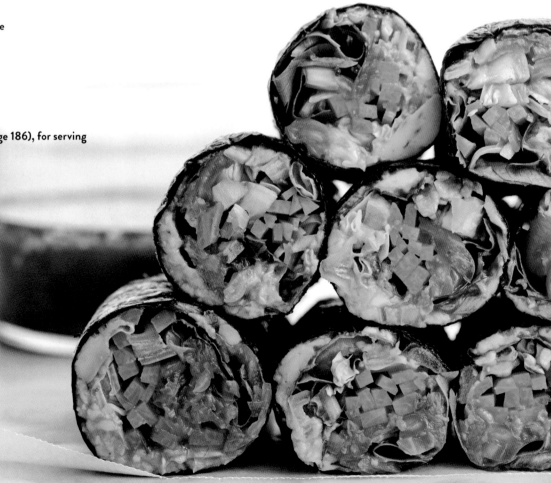

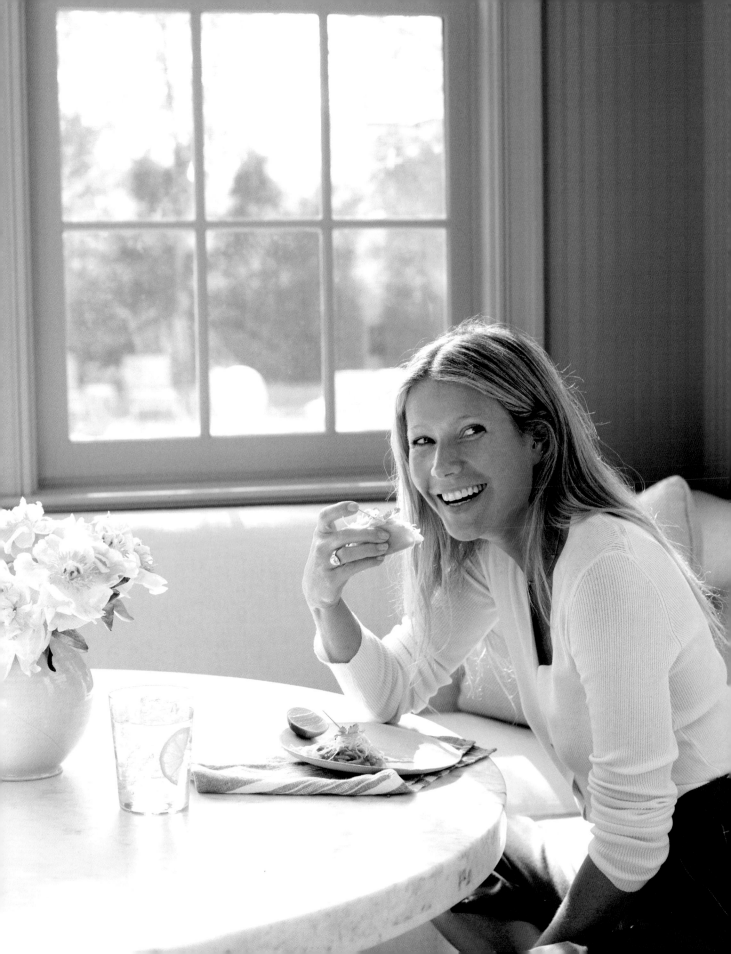

A LITTLE MORE FILLING

Despite what you may have heard, clean eating isn't all green juice and sad vegan food. While I tend to gravitate toward lighter salads and wraps for lunch, when it comes to dinner, I'm definitely a turkey burger/spaghetti and meatballs/roast chicken and potatoes kind of girl. I want something that will fill me up and warm me from the inside out; something cooked with love and layered with flavor. If I'm not doing a January kickoff cleanse or testing detox recipes, I typically eat whatever I want at dinner. But with no nightshades (bye, potatoes), gluten (adios, burger bun), or dairy (sayonara, Parmesan), so many of those classic comfort foods can seem totally off-limits. So I've made it my mission to develop clean versions of some of my favorites. You'll find a killer turkey burger wrapped in lettuce and piled high with avocado, pickle, and creamy aquafaba; lemony turkey meatballs slow-simmered in "nomato" sauce; meat loaf; chicken tacos; and more. These delicious and totally satisfying dishes never feel like a compromise. They leave me—and my French fry–loving friends and family—feeling full and happy, and I suspect they'll do the same for you and yours.

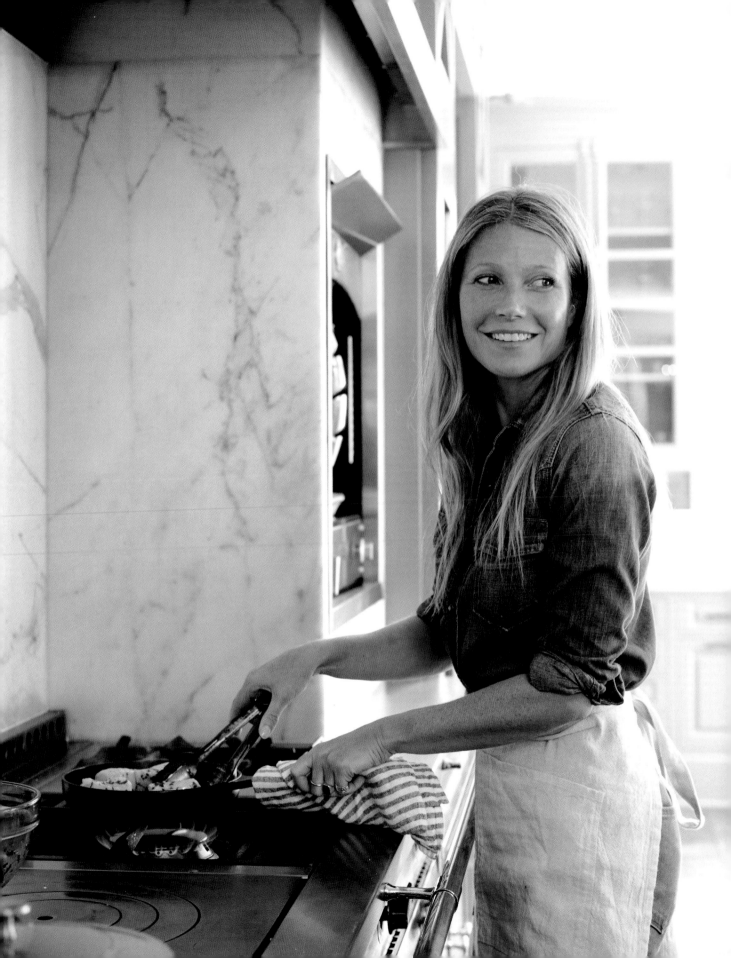

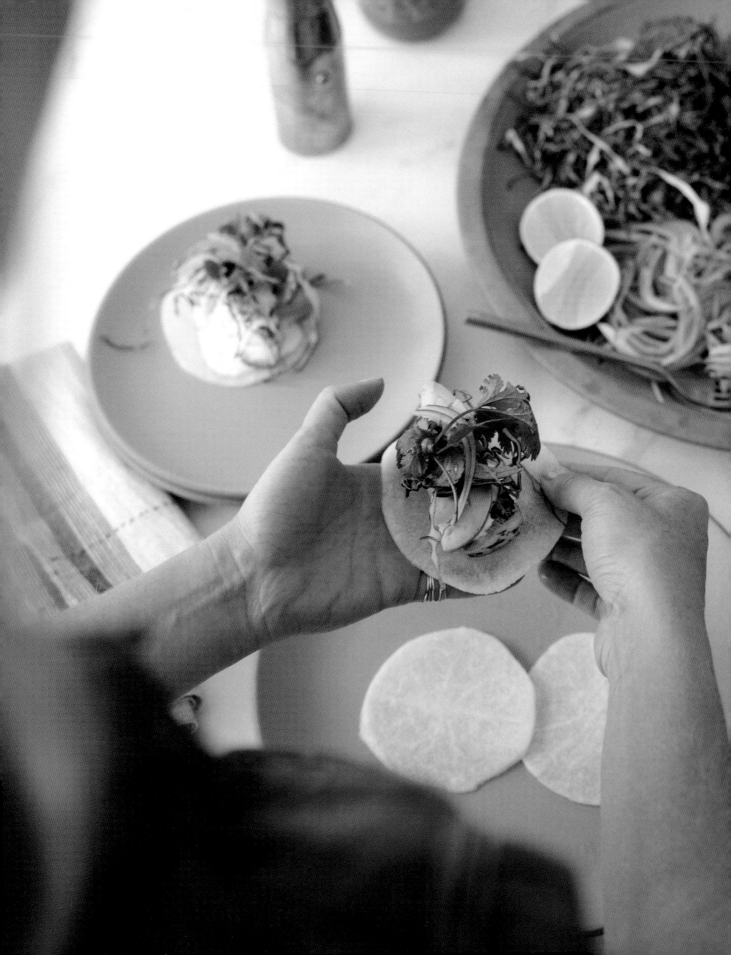

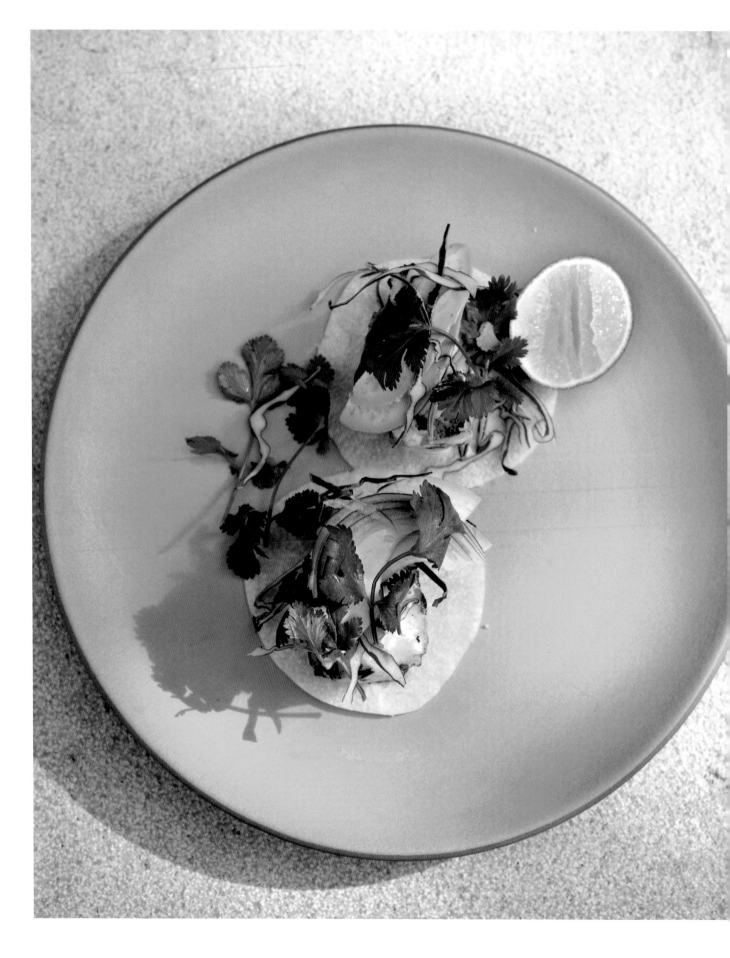

Fish Tacos on Jicama "Tortillas"

Serves 2

These grain-free, gluten-free, etc.-free taco shells are legit brilliant. I first heard about using jicama as a tortilla replacement from a friend of a friend who'd recently returned from a trip to Tulum, Mexico. Let's just say my (healthy) taco life has been made infinitely better.

FOR THE FISH:

½ pound halibut fillet, skin and bones removed

2 tablespoons olive oil

2 tablespoons chopped fresh cilantro

Juice of ½ lime

⅛ teaspoon ground cumin

Flaky sea salt

FOR THE TACOS:

1 small jicama (about 5 inches in diameter), peeled

½ cup shredded cabbage

Juice of ½ lime

Kosher salt

Sliced red onion

½ avocado, thinly sliced

Drizzle of Aquafaba Crema (page 180)

Fresh cilantro leaves

Lime wedges, for serving

To make the fish, cut the halibut into 4 equal strips. Place in a bowl and toss with the olive oil, cilantro, lime juice, cumin, and a large pinch of flaky salt. Cover and set aside to marinate for a few minutes.

To make the tacos, use a jumbo mandoline to slice four ⅛-inch-thick "tortillas" from the jicama. (If you don't have a jumbo mandoline, do this carefully with a sharp knife.)

In a small bowl, toss the cabbage with the lime juice and a pinch of kosher salt and set aside.

Heat a small nonstick pan over medium-high heat. Add the halibut and cook for about 2 minutes on each side, or until just cooked through.

Place one piece of fish on each jicama "tortilla" and top with the shredded cabbage, red onion, and avocado. Drizzle with aquafaba crema and finish with cilantro.

Serve with lime wedges on the side for squeezing.

Faux Meat Beet Tacos

VEGAN

Serves 2

Legumes can be a nice source of protein, especially if you're trying to eat a plant-based diet. But they can be difficult for some of us to digest. Enter this beet taco recipe. Beets are earthy and have a minerality to them that means they can be a great stand-in for meat or beans. (Don't knock it till you try it.) And don't worry about letting the beets brown on the stovetop for a while—the flavor gets much deeper and richer if you let them caramelize nicely.

FOR THE FILLING:

2 tablespoons olive oil

½ white onion, finely diced

2 garlic cloves, minced

¼ teaspoon ground coriander

½ teaspoon ground cumin

¼ teaspoon chili flakes (optional)

½ teaspoon kosher salt

¾ cup finely diced Roasted Beets (page 198)

FOR THE TACOS:

4 small grain-free tortillas (I like coconut and cassava flour tortillas)

½ avocado, sliced

Pickled Radishes (page 208)

Aquafaba Crema (page 180)

½ cup shredded cabbage

Lime wedges, for serving

Fresh cilantro leaves, for garnish

To make the filling, in a large sauté pan, heat the olive oil over medium heat. Add the onion, garlic, and spices and cook, stirring, for 5 to 7 minutes, until the onion and garlic soften and begin to caramelize. Add the beets and cook for 7 to 10 minutes more, until they are nicely browned.

To assemble the tacos, pile one-quarter of the beet mixture into each tortilla, then top with a slice of avocado, a few pickles, a drizzle of crema, and a bit of cabbage. Finish with a squeeze of lime juice and a few cilantro leaves and serve.

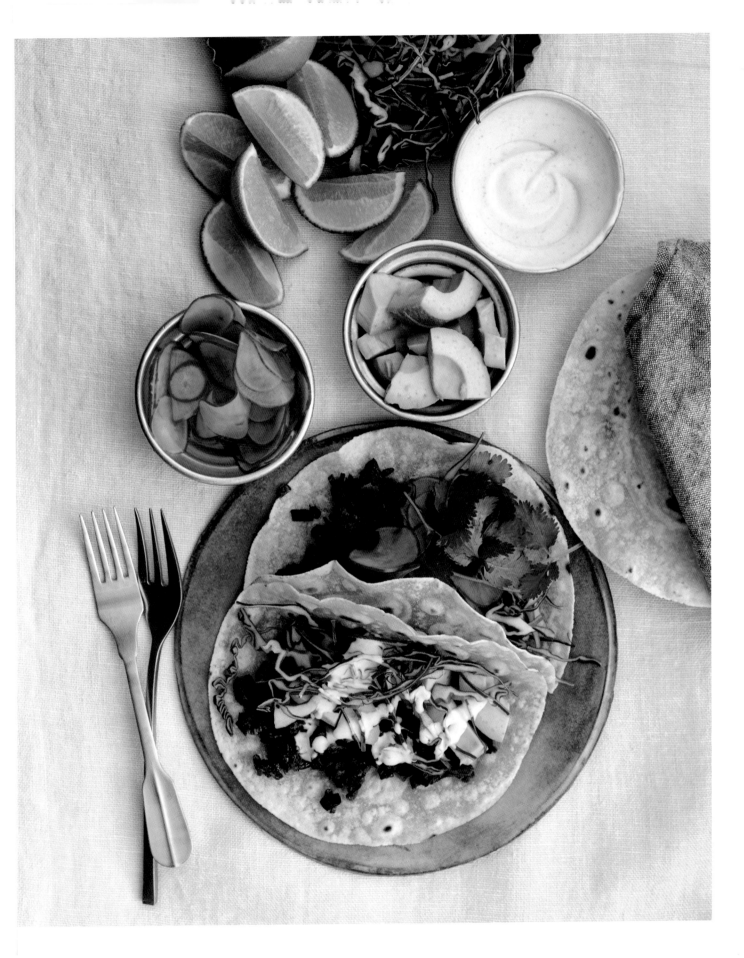

Zoodle Chow Mein

QUICK

Serves 2

My whole family loves chow mein, but the classic recipe, made with wheat noodles and tons of oil, is not exactly "clean." Thanks to the trusty zucchini noodle, or "zoodle," this version scratches the Chinese takeout itch, minus the sodium bomb.

1 boneless, skinless chicken breast

Kosher salt

4 tablespoons olive oil

½ large yellow onion, thinly sliced

2 shiitake, oyster, or maitake mushrooms, thinly sliced

1 garlic clove, grated

½ teaspoon grated fresh ginger

1 large or 2 small zucchini, spiralized

1 teaspoon toasted sesame oil

2 tablespoons coconut aminos

Kosher salt

Cut the chicken breast into ½-inch-thick slices, then cut the slices into 2-inch pieces. Season generously with salt.

In a large nonstick pan or wok, heat 2 tablespoons of the olive oil over medium-high heat. Add the onion and cook, stirring, for 2 minutes, or until beginning to brown. Add the mushrooms and cook, stirring often, for 1 minute.

Push the onion and mushrooms to the side of the pan and add the remaining 2 tablespoons olive oil and the chicken to the empty side. Cook until the chicken is starting to brown on the first side, then flip and cook for another minute or two, until almost cooked through.

Stir in the mushroom-onion mixture, then add the garlic and ginger and sauté for 30 seconds, adding a little water if the pan looks dry.

Add the zucchini noodles, sesame oil, and coconut aminos and season everything with a big pinch of salt. Toss to combine, taste and adjust the seasoning, and serve.

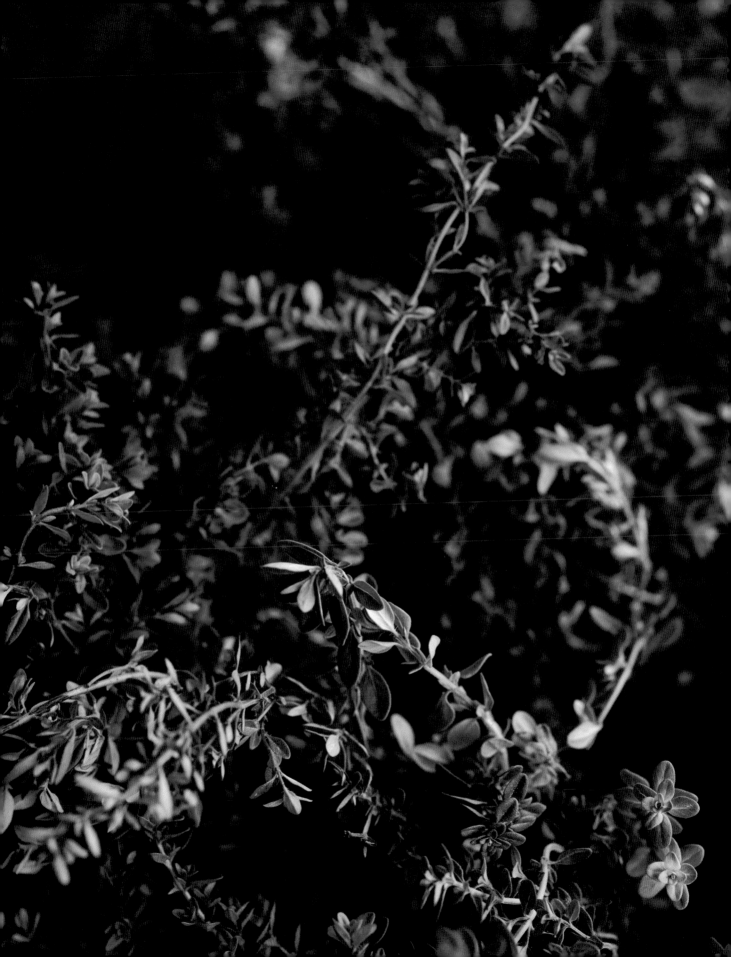

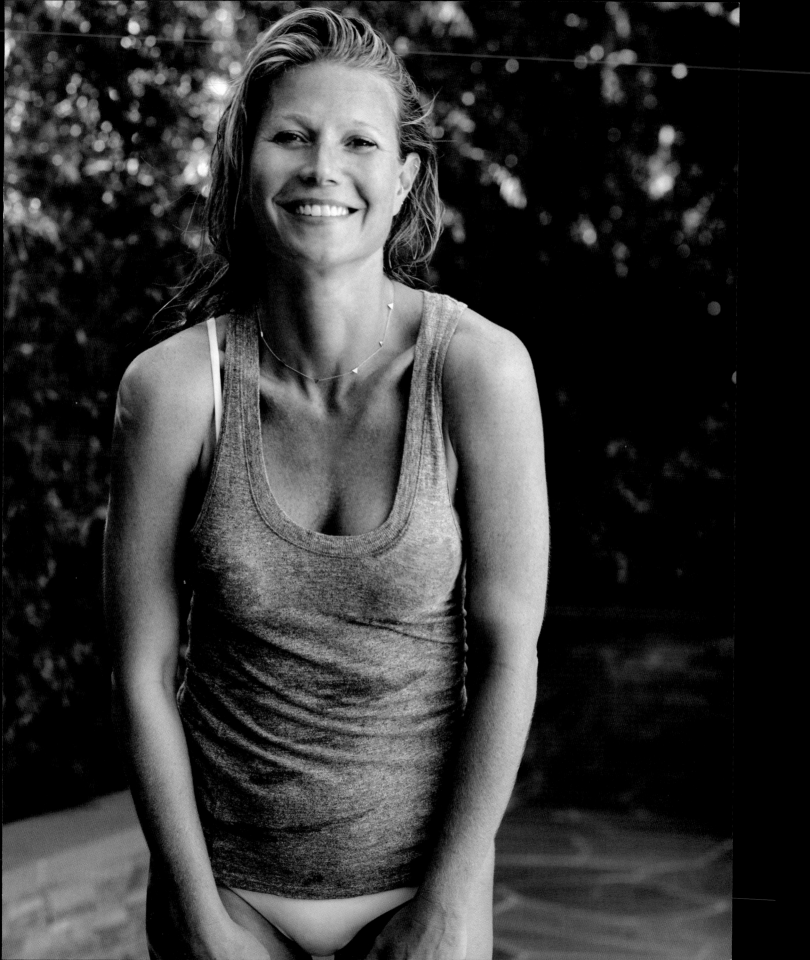

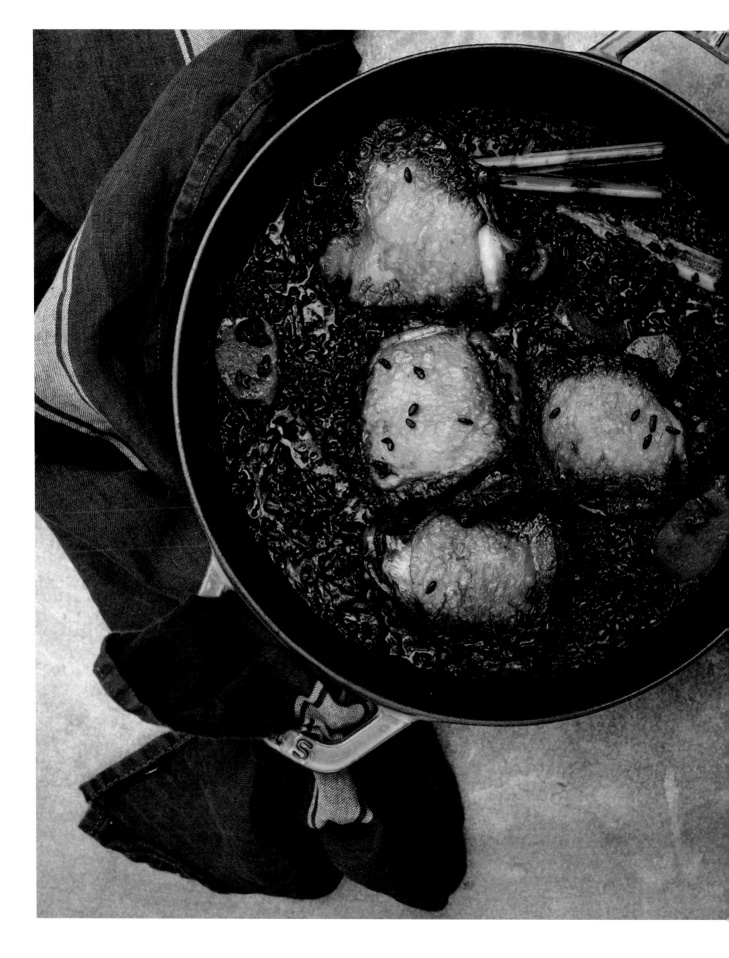

Black Rice with Braised Chicken Thighs

Serves 2

One of my favorites for entertaining, this dish is both incredibly delicious and gorgeous. As the chicken simmers in the gingery, lemongrassy, coconutty black rice, it takes on tons of flavor and an intense purple hue. Eat this plain, curled up in front of the TV, or serve it to guests with a simple salad or grilled vegetable on the side.

4 bone-in, skin-on chicken thighs

¼ teaspoon kosher salt, plus more for seasoning the chicken

1 teaspoon coconut oil

1 (2-inch) piece fresh ginger, peeled and sliced

3 large garlic cloves, sliced

⅔ cup black rice

1½ cups water

½ cup full-fat coconut milk

1 lemongrass stalk, outside layer peeled off, smashed with the side of a knife

Season the chicken thighs generously with salt on both sides.

In a 12-inch braiser or sauté pan with a lid, melt the coconut oil over medium-high heat. Add the chicken thighs, skin-side down, and sear until very nicely browned. Flip and cook until browned on the second side, about 5 minutes each side. Transfer to a plate and set aside.

Add the ginger and garlic and cook, stirring, for 30 seconds, or until fragrant but not browned.

Add the rice and give it a stir, coating each grain with the oil.

Add the water, coconut milk, lemongrass, and salt. Bring the mixture to a simmer, then return the chicken thighs to the pan, skin-side up, and cover. Reduce the heat to the lowest setting and simmer gently for 45 minutes.

Divide rice and serve with two thighs.

Kitchari

VEGAN

Serves 2

This humble dish is so warming and nourishing. In Ayurvedic medicine, *kitchari* is a balancing staple (see page 251 for more on Ayurveda from Dr. Aruna). I enjoy it for breakfast, but you can have it any time of day. It's pretty delicious with a dollop of unsweetened coconut yogurt swirled in, too.

⅓ cup moong dal (split mung beans)

¼ cup basmati rice

1 tablespoon coconut oil

1 tablespoon curry powder

½ teaspoon kosher salt

2 cups water

½ cup roughly chopped fresh cilantro

Put the beans and rice in a bowl and rinse with cool running water. Drain and repeat once or twice more.

In a medium saucepan, melt the coconut oil over medium heat. Add the curry powder, beans, rice, and salt. Cook, stirring, for a couple of minutes, then add the water. Bring to a boil, then cover and reduce the heat to low. Cook for 20 minutes, undisturbed, until thick and creamy.

Divide the kitchari between two bowls. Garnish with the cilantro.

FISH EN PAPILLOTE, 2 WAYS

Cooking fish in parchment paper, or as the French say, *en papillote*, is cool for many reasons—wonderful flavor, moist fish, fun presentation—but I'd have to say the biggest draw is the easy cleanup. Everything cooks in one little parchment parcel, making it the most elegant one-pot dinner.

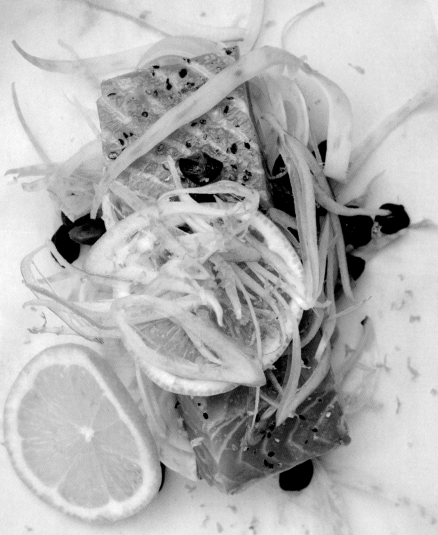

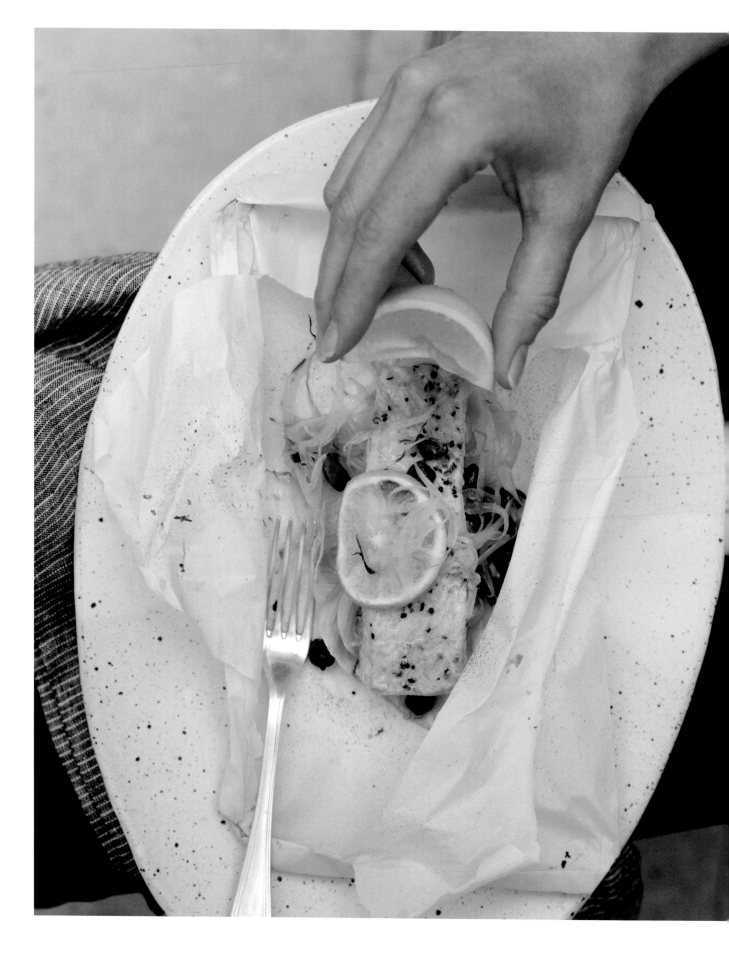

Mediterranean Salmon en Papillote

QUICK

Serves 2

It's hard to go wrong with fennel, lemon, and capers, especially when you throw salmon in the mix. This is a foolproof method regardless of your dietary philosophy.

2 (6-ounce) pieces salmon, skin removed

Flaky sea salt and cracked black pepper

1 small fennel bulb, thinly sliced

1 small shallot, thinly sliced

4 lemon slices

2 teaspoons capers

½ teaspoon grated lemon zest

Olive oil

A dash of Aleppo pepper (optional)

Preheat the oven to 400°F. Lay out two 9x11-inch sheets of parchment paper on a flat surface.

Season the salmon fillets generously with salt and black pepper and place one in the lower third section of each parchment sheet. Divide the fennel, shallot, lemon slices, capers, and lemon zest evenly between the fillets.

Drizzle a little olive oil (about 1 tablespoon total) over each and sprinkle with Aleppo pepper, if desired.

Fold the top half of the parchment paper over the fish to make a rectangle. Starting on one side, crimp the edges together tightly so no liquid can escape and the contents are completely enclosed. Repeat with the other two sides, then place the parcels on a baking sheet and bake for 12 to 15 minutes, depending on the thickness of the fillets.

Transfer the parcels to individual plates. Carefully cut open the parchment paper (the steam inside is hot) and serve.

Halibut en Papillote with Lemon, Mushrooms & Toasted Sesame Oil

QUICK

Serves 2

As far as I'm concerned, almost anything with toasted sesame oil is going to be good, and that's certainly true of this ginger-scented halibut-and-mushroom parcel. Like the previous papillote recipe, this serves two, but could be easily scaled up for a bigger crowd. (It seems like all my friends want to come over when I'm making it.)

2 medium shiitake, oyster, or maitake mushrooms, thinly sliced

2 (6-ounce) halibut fillets, skin removed

Flaky sea salt and cracked black pepper

½ teaspoon grated lemon zest

½ teaspoon grated fresh ginger

2 scallions, thinly sliced

1 teaspoon coconut aminos

½ teaspoon toasted sesame oil, plus more for drizzling

4 lemon slices

Preheat the oven to 400°F. Lay out two 9x11-inch sheets of parchment paper on a flat surface.

Place the sliced mushrooms in the lower third of each parchment sheet. Season the halibut fillets generously with salt and pepper and place them on top of the mushrooms.

Divide the lemon zest, ginger, scallions, coconut aminos, sesame oil, and lemon slices evenly between the fillets.

Fold the top half of the parchment paper over the fish to make a rectangle. Starting on one side, crimp the edges together tightly so no liquid can escape and the contents are completely enclosed. Repeat with the other two edges, then place the parcels on a baking sheet and bake for 12 to 15 minutes, depending on the thickness of the fillets.

Transfer the parcels to individual plates. Carefully cut open the parchment paper (the steam inside is hot) and serve.

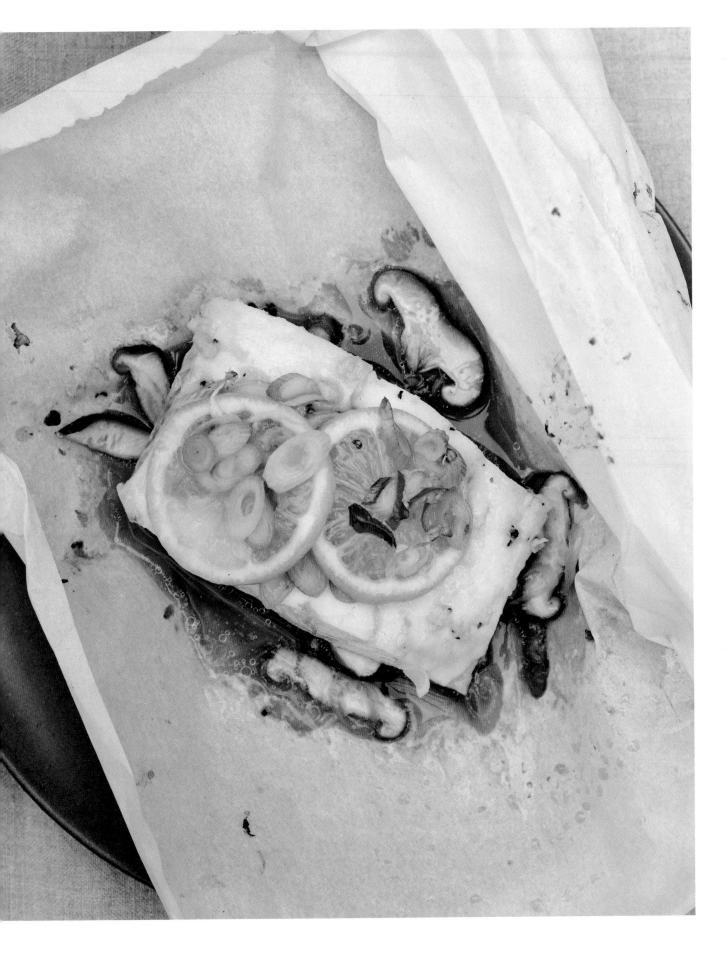

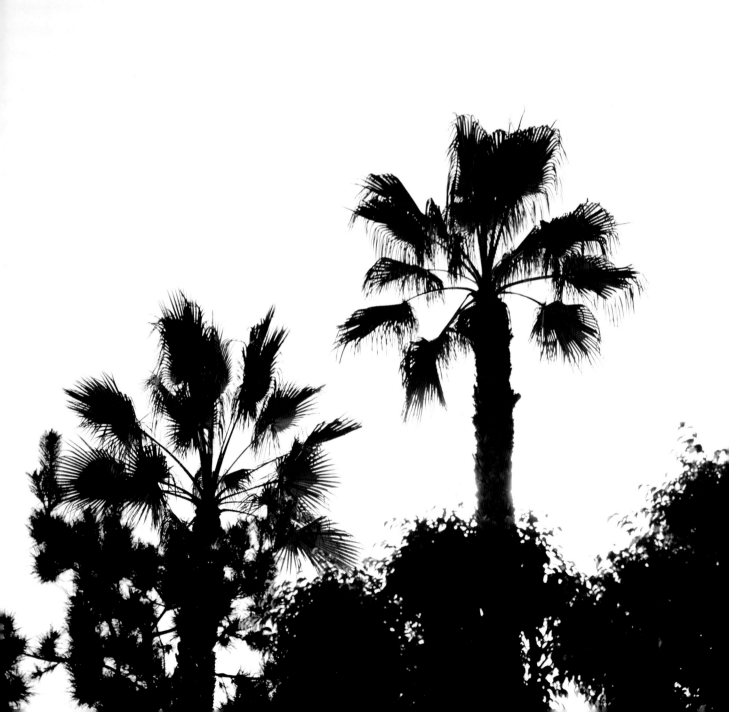

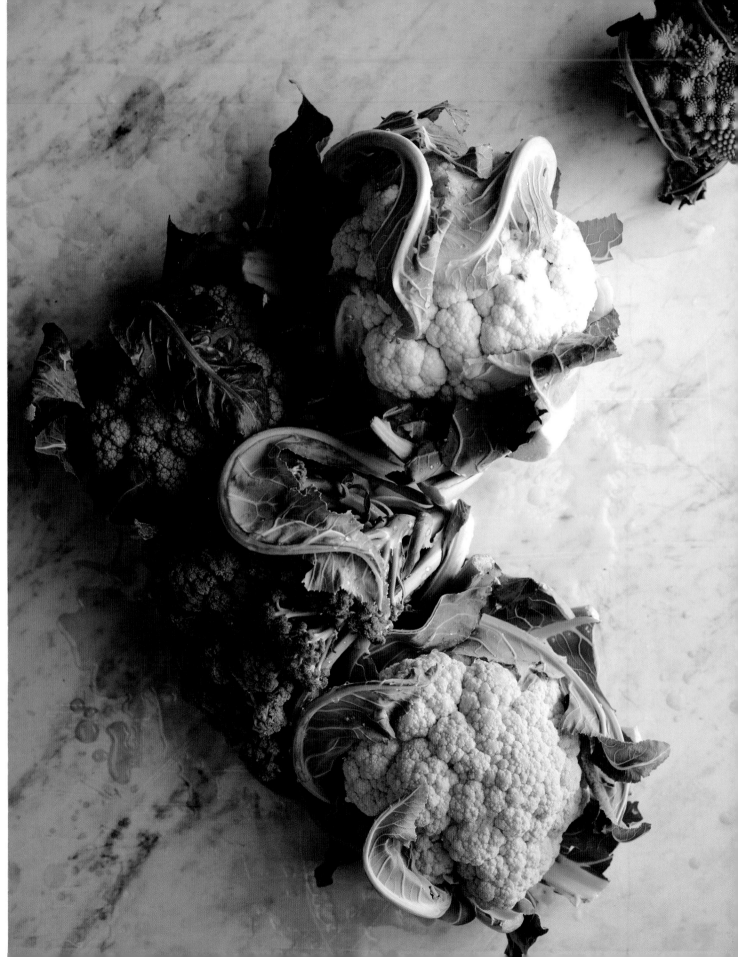

Sheet Pan Chicken with Broccolini & Radicchio

Serves 2

Italian food is easily the thing I miss most when I'm eating really clean (Parm, prosciutto, pasta—I'm looking at you). This sheet pan dinner is great because you get to enjoy a lot of those flavors, but in a much lighter dish. If you don't care for the bitter flavor of radicchio, you could try using Tuscan kale instead.

1 pound boneless, skinless chicken thighs, cut into 2-inch pieces

1 lemon, thinly sliced

2 tablespoons Parsley Salsa Verde (page 183), plus more for serving

Kosher salt

1 bunch of Broccolini, ends trimmed, split lengthwise

½ head of radicchio, cut into 4 wedges through the core

6 garlic cloves, smashed

Olive oil

Flaky sea salt

Preheat the oven to 425°F. Line a baking sheet with parchment paper.

In a large bowl, toss together the chicken, lemon slices, salsa verde, and a generous pinch of kosher salt. Spread the mixture over the prepared baking sheet and roast for 10 minutes.

In a separate large bowl, toss together the Broccolini, radicchio, and garlic with a glug of olive oil and a generous pinch of kosher salt. Add the vegetable mixture to the baking sheet with the chicken and lemon, toss to combine, and bake for 5 to 8 minutes more, or until the Broccolini is crispy and the radicchio is wilted.

Finish with flaky salt and drizzle with salsa verde before serving.

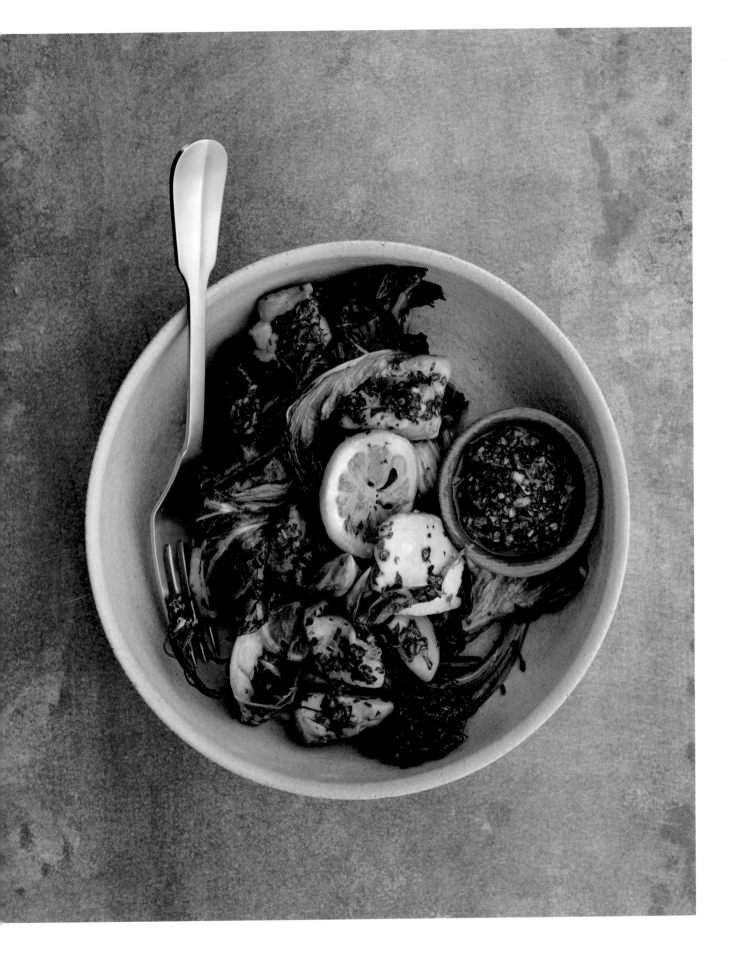

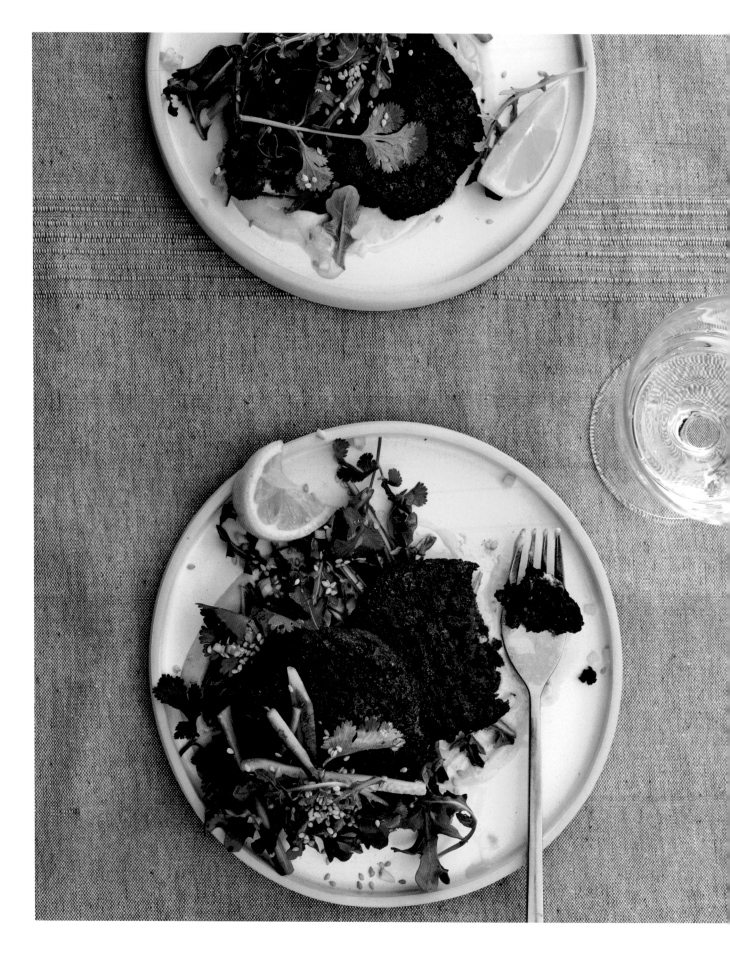

Beet Falafel Sliders

VEGAN

Serves 4

Falafel flavors are decidedly rich and savory, yet still so fresh-tasting with all that parsley. These are a fun take on the classic, and the beets add a subtle sweetness, not to mention a beautiful color. My kids eat them with hummus, but they're also delicious with tahini dressing.

1 cup chopped Roasted Beets (page 198)

1 cup chickpeas

1 large handful of parsley (just shy of 1 cup)

4 garlic cloves

¼ red onion, chopped

1 teaspoon ground cumin

½ teaspoon kosher salt

¼ cup chickpea flour

2 tablespoons olive oil

1 cup baby arugula

¼ cup fresh cilantro leaves

1 tablespoon fresh lemon juice

Flaky sea salt

Tahini Dressing (page 189), for serving

Preheat the oven to 425°F. Place an unlined baking sheet in the oven to preheat.

In a food processor, combine the beets, chickpeas, parsley, garlic, onion, cumin, kosher salt, and chickpea flour and pulse for a few minutes until well combined. Divide the mixture into 8 portions and form them into even patties, 2 to 3 inches in diameter.

Carefully remove the hot baking sheet from the oven and brush it with the olive oil. Lay the falafel patties on the baking sheet and bake for about 10 minutes. Flip the falafel and bake for 10 minutes more.

Meanwhile, in a small bowl, toss the arugula and cilantro with the lemon juice and a pinch of flaky salt.

To serve, lay two beet burgers on each plate. Drizzle with dressing and top each with half the arugula salad.

White Bean & Zucchini Burgers

VEGAN

Serves 4

Typically, I loathe bean burgers—more often than not, they're bland and stodgy. These burgers, however, are different. The texture of grated zucchini and millet becomes so pleasantly crispy, and then there's the schmear of lemony garlic aquafaba and a pickled onion to boot.

2 tablespoons olive oil, plus more as needed

2 medium leeks, washed well and diced

8 crimini mushrooms, diced

8 garlic cloves, minced

Zest of 1 lemon

1 cup canned cannellini beans, drained

1 cup cooked millet, cooled

1 cup grated zucchini

2 teaspoons kosher salt

2 cups baby kale

Pickled Red Onions (page 206)

Lemony Garlic Aquafaba Sauce (page 179)

In a sauté pan, heat the olive oil over medium-high heat. Add the leeks, mushrooms, and garlic and cook, stirring, until caramelized, about 7 minutes. Remove from the heat, add the lemon zest, and set aside to cool.

Meanwhile, in a medium bowl, mash together the beans, millet, zucchini, and salt. Once the vegetable mixture has cooled, add it to the bowl and stir well to combine. Form the mixture into 4 patties.

In a nonstick skillet, heat a few tablespoons of olive oil over medium-high heat. Add the patties and cook for 3 to 5 minutes on each side, until crispy and browned, being careful not to break them on the flip.

Meanwhile, in a small bowl, toss the baby kale with pickled onions.

Serve the kale and onions alongside the bean burgers and lemony garlic aquafaba.

Five-Spice Salmon Burgers

QUICK

Makes 6 burgers

A riff on the salmon burgers from *It's All Good*, these are soy-free but don't sacrifice anything on taste. The Chinese five-spice powder (usually a mix of star anise, cloves, cinnamon, Sichuan peppercorn, and fennel) is clutch.

1½ pounds salmon, skin removed, cut into 1-inch pieces

4 scallions, thinly sliced

1 garlic clove, minced

1 (2-inch) piece fresh ginger, peeled and minced

½ teaspoon Chinese five-spice powder

2 tablespoons coconut aminos

½ teaspoon kosher salt

½ teaspoon toasted sesame oil

Place the salmon pieces on a plate and freeze for about 10 minutes, until very cold but not frozen. In batches, transfer the salmon to a food processor and pulse until it's well minced but not so much that it breaks down into a paste, about ten 1-second pulses. Transfer the salmon to a large bowl.

Combine the remaining ingredients in the food processor and process until very smooth, about 1 minute. Add to the bowl with the salmon and use a fork, spatula, or clean hands to thoroughly incorporate all the ingredients. Either cook right away or cover and refrigerate for up to 2 days.

Form the salmon mixture into 6 equal patties. Heat a grill pan over medium-high heat. When the pan is hot (but not smoking), add the salmon patties and cook for about 3 minutes on each side.

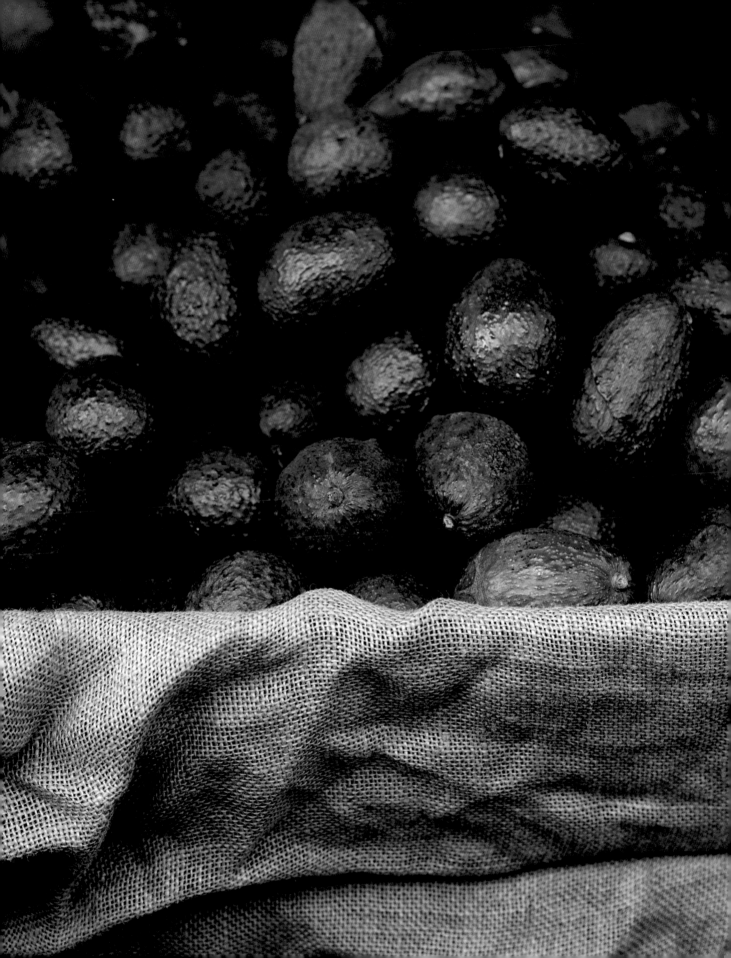

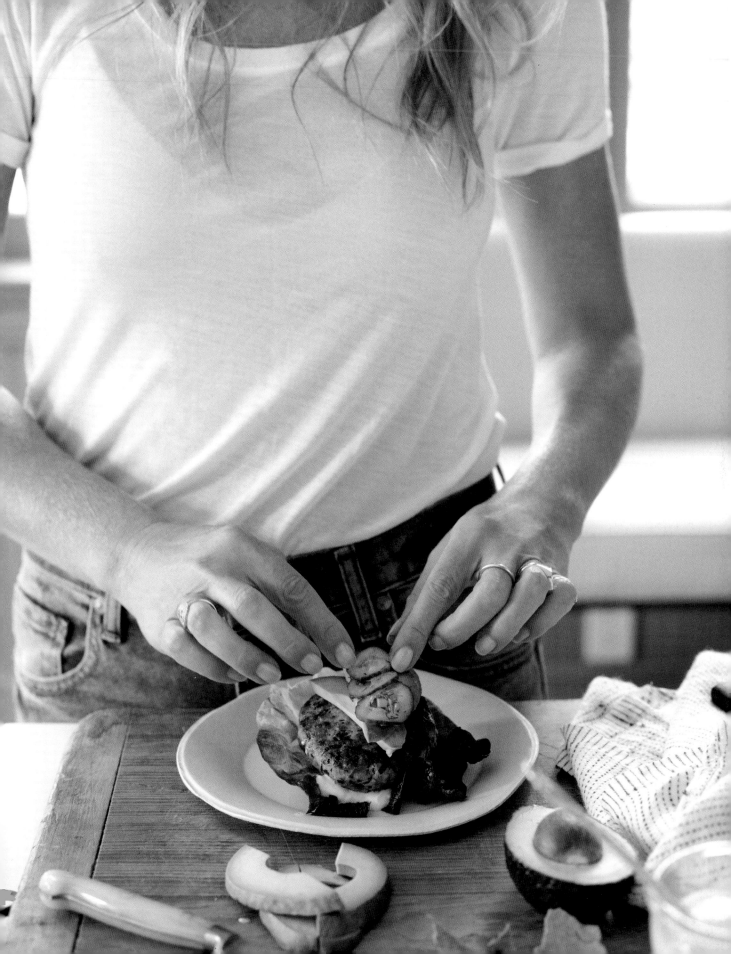

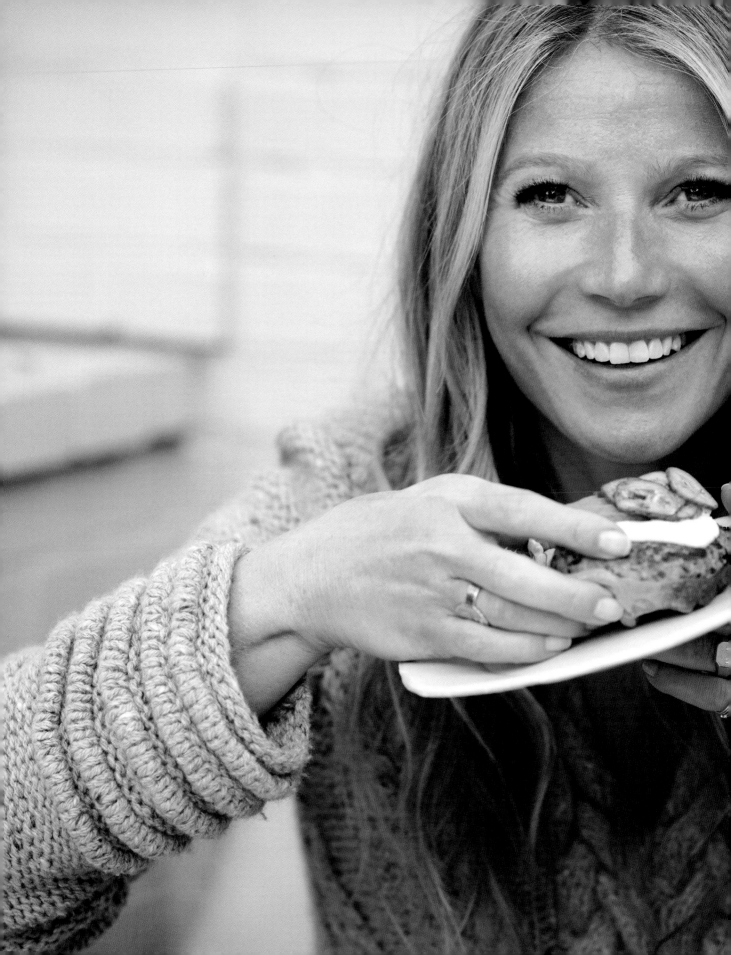

Turkey Burgers

QUICK

Serves 4

At the end of the day, I'm a burger kind of woman, and this one hits all the marks: grilled, savory, herbed patty; cool, lemony aquafaba; crisp lettuce; creamy avocado; and a little crunch and tang from a pickle. This does not feel like detox food, that's for sure.

1 pound dark meat ground turkey

4 garlic cloves, grated

½ cup chopped fresh cilantro

2 tablespoons chopped fresh mint

½ teaspoon ground cumin

½ teaspoon kosher salt

Zest of 1 lime

Olive oil

Red-leaf lettuce, for serving

½ avocado, sliced

Pickled Cucumbers (page 209)

Lemony Garlic Aquafaba Sauce (page 179)

In a medium bowl, combine the ground turkey, garlic, cilantro, mint, cumin, salt, and lime zest and mix well. Shape the mixture into 4 equal patties.

Heat a grill pan over medium-high heat. Brush the pan with a little olive oil, then add the patties and cook for a few minutes on each side.

To serve, wrap a turkey burger in lettuce and top with sliced avocado, pickles, and lemony garlic aquafaba.

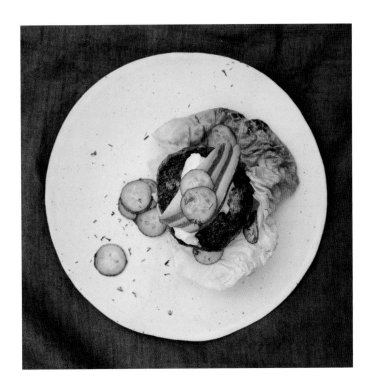

Italian Braised Chicken

Serves 2 or 3

When I'm flipping through recipes in the realm of clean eating, I'm often thinking, *But those are just raw vegetables…*And sure, that can be great, and sometimes when I'm eating clean I weirdly do end up craving snap peas and radishes more than my Gouda and baguette. But what I really want is comfort food that is also totally clean, for those days I just really need it. Enter nomato sauce. I took inspiration from a tomato-y braised chicken a friend made me, but I tried it with nomato sauce, and it really worked. We've been eating it over brown rice pasta, but you can try it with lentil or chickpea pasta or over cauliflower rice.

3 tablespoons olive oil

2 bone-in, skin-on chicken breasts

Kosher salt

½ white onion, diced

2 garlic cloves, grated

2 thyme sprigs

2 cups Nomato Sauce (page 191)

12 ounces brown rice spaghetti

A few torn fresh basil leaves, to garnish

Flaky sea salt and cracked black pepper

Preheat the oven to 350°F.

In a Dutch oven, heat the olive oil over medium-high heat. Season the chicken generously with kosher salt. Add it to the pan, skin-side down, and sear for a few minutes, just until nicely browned, then flip and do the same on the other side.

Remove the chicken from the pan and set it aside on a plate. Reduce the heat to medium-low and add the onion, garlic, and thyme. Cook until lightly caramelized, scraping up all the browned bits from the bottom of the pan, then add the nomato sauce and return the browned chicken breasts to the pan. Cover the pot and transfer to the oven. Braise for about 1½ hours, or until the chicken is tender.

Meanwhile, cook the spaghetti according to the package directions.

Remove and discard the thyme sprigs. Remove the chicken and let cool slightly, then shred the meat and stir it back into the sauce. Add the pasta to the pot with the chicken and sauce and toss to combine.

Garnish with the basil, finish with flaky salt and cracked pepper, and serve.

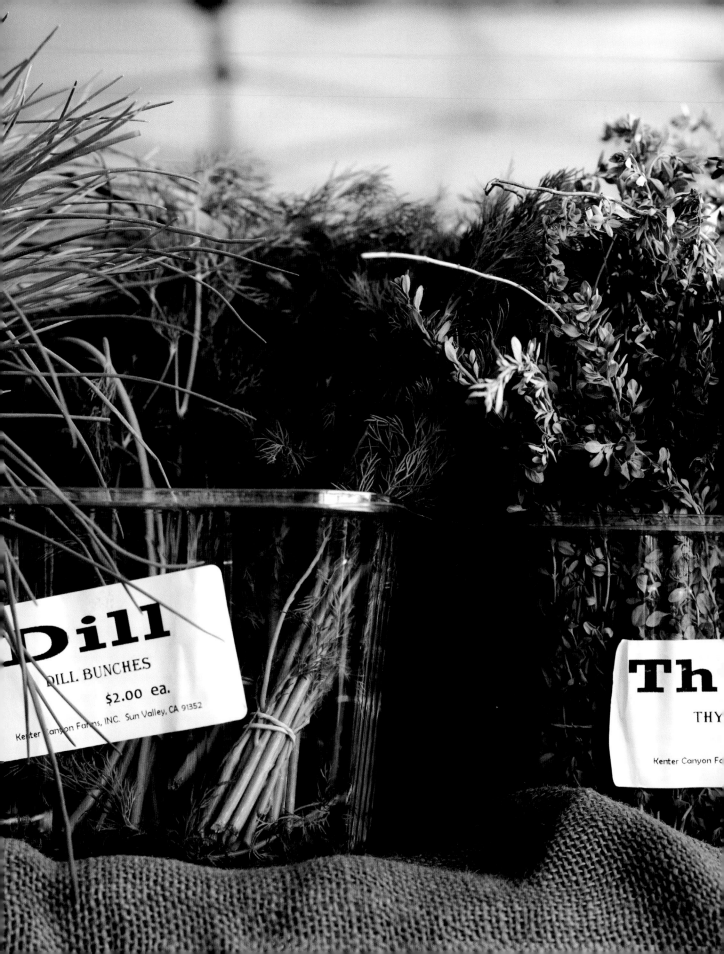

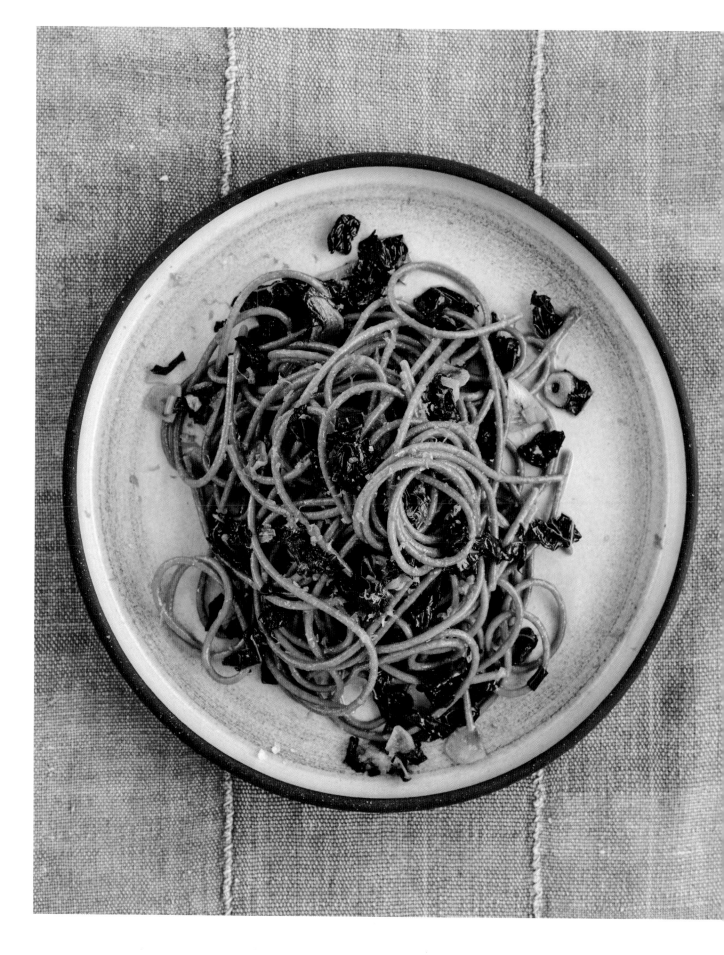

Kale Aglio e Olio

QUICK / VEGAN

Serves 2

I enjoy making *aglio e olio* (pasta with garlic and olive oil), and adding kale to it is a good way to sneak in some extra greens. (If you sprinkle some Parm on top for your kids, they might go nuts for it as well.) You can use brown rice pasta here if you prefer, or go for lentil or chickpea pasta for a bit of extra protein.

8 ounces lentil spaghetti

¼ cup olive oil, plus more if needed

6 garlic cloves, thinly sliced

3 anchovy fillets (optional)

1 bunch of black kale, stemmed and sliced into thin ribbons (about 2 cups)

Zest of ½ lemon

Flaky sea salt

Chili flakes (optional)

Bring a large pot of water to a boil. Add the spaghetti and cook for a little bit less time than the box suggests so it will stay al dente. Drain and rinse with cold water for a couple of minutes. Set aside.

In a large, shallow sauté pan, heat the olive oil over medium-high heat. Add the garlic and anchovy (if using) and cook, stirring frequently and making sure nothing burns, for about 1 minute. Add the kale and cook for another minute, then add the lemon zest and spaghetti and toss everything together. Drizzle in a little extra olive oil, if needed.

Divide the pasta between two bowls. Finish with flaky salt and chili flakes, if desired, and serve.

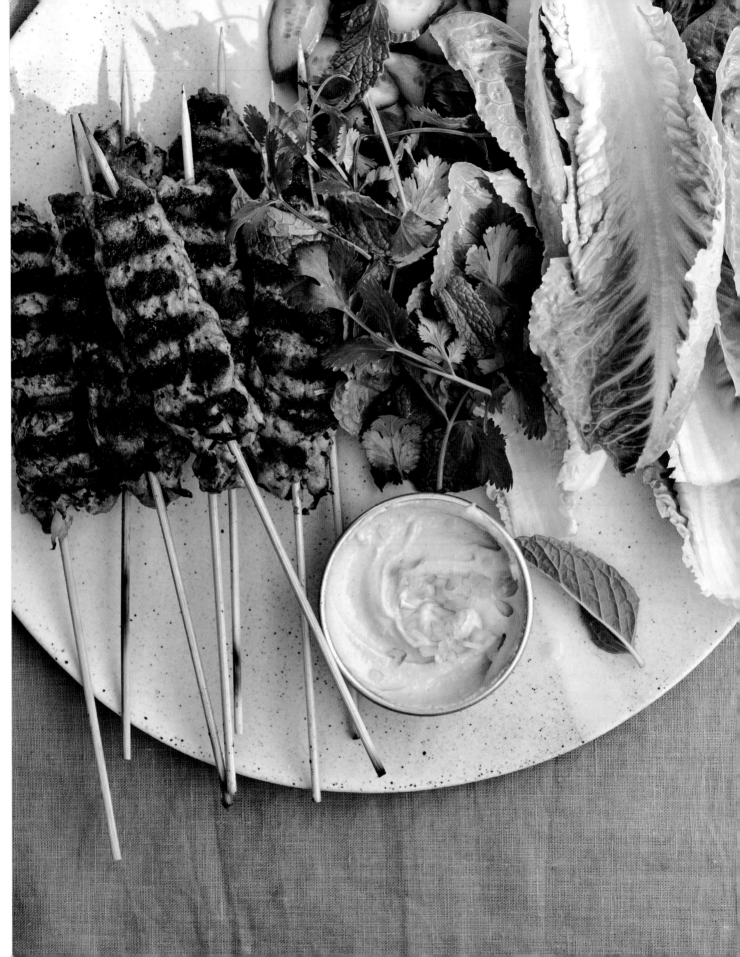

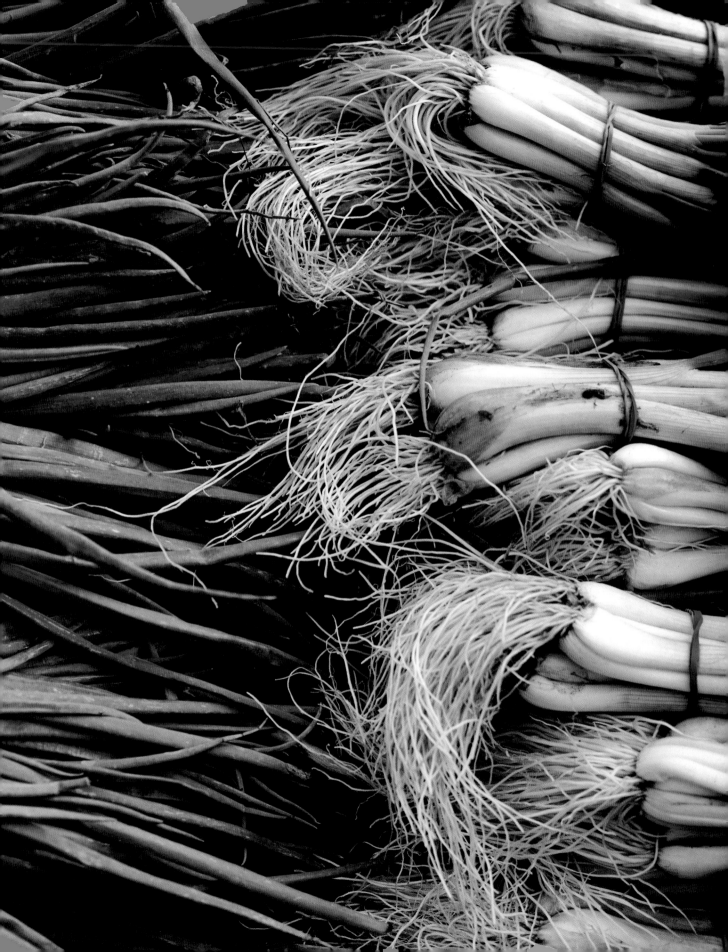

Chicken & Zucchini Kefta

Serves 2

Packed with flavor and fresh ingredients, these chicken kebabs feel like the opposite of a sacrifice, and are a summer BBQ staple. If skewering sounds like too much work, form these into little meatballs or burgers instead. And don't skip the tahini sauce—it really ties everything together.

FOR THE KEBABS:

1 medium zucchini, grated

1½ teaspoons kosher salt

1 pound ground dark meat chicken

2 scallions, thinly sliced (about ⅓ cup)

2 tablespoons chopped fresh cilantro

⅓ cup chopped fresh mint

3 garlic cloves, finely chopped

2 tablespoons very finely chopped fresh ginger

1 teaspoon ground cumin

1 teaspoon ground coriander

½ teaspoon ground cinnamon

2 tablespoons tahini

Olive oil

TO SERVE:

Whole romaine or butter lettuce leaves

½ cucumber, sliced

16 cilantro sprigs

1 cup whole mint leaves

Tahini Dressing (page 189)

To make the kebabs, soak 12 small wooden skewers in water for 20 minutes.

In a small bowl, combine the zucchini and ½ teaspoon of the salt and let sit for 5 minutes. Squeeze out as much liquid as possible.

In a large bowl, combine the zucchini, chicken, scallions, cilantro, mint, garlic, ginger, cumin, coriander, cinnamon, and tahini. Divide the mixture into 12 portions, then, with damp hands, shape each portion around a skewer.

Heat a grill or grill pan to medium-high. Brush the kebabs with a bit of olive oil, then grill for 8 to 10 minutes on each side, until cooked through.

Place the kebabs on a platter with whole lettuce leaves, the cucumber, cilantro, and mint. Serve with the dressing.

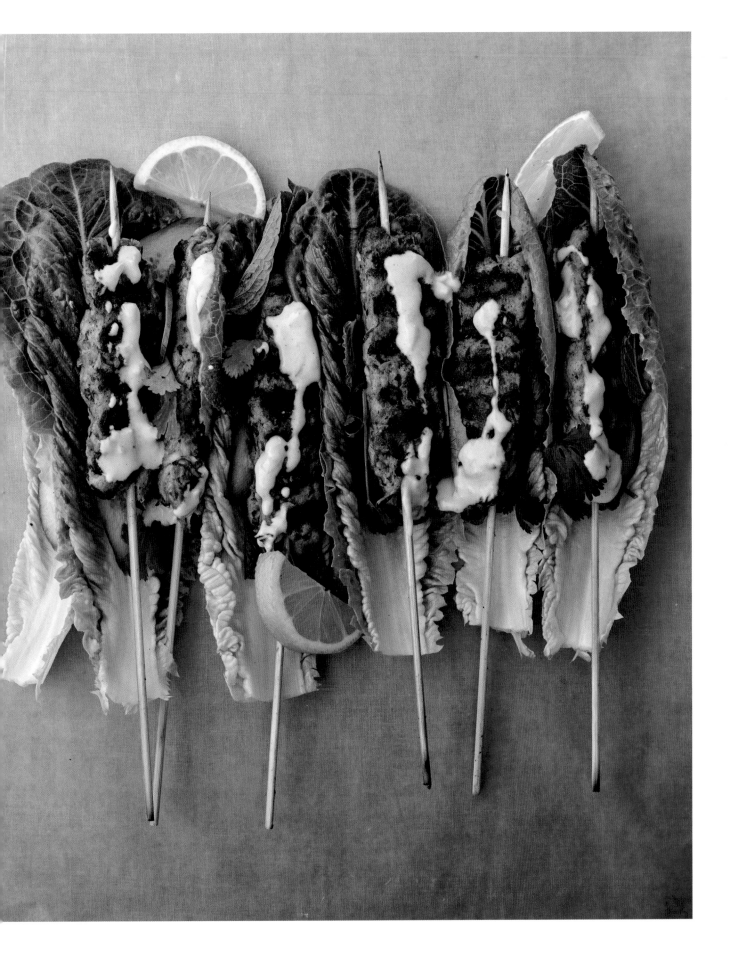

Braised Mexican Nomato Chicken

Serves 2

I'm addicted to my Braised Mexican Chicken recipe, which you can find on goop.com, but when I'm cutting out nightshades, that tomato-based sauce is, unfortunately, off-limits. Here's the super-easy clean version—welcome at taco night with the fam.

1 boneless, skinless chicken breast

Kosher salt

1 tablespoon olive oil

2 garlic cloves, minced

2 tablespoons finely chopped fresh cilantro (stems and leaves)

¼ teaspoon ground cumin

1 cup Nomato Sauce (page 191)

Season the chicken breast generously with salt.

In a 2-quart saucepan, heat the olive oil over medium-low heat. Add the garlic, cilantro, and cumin and cook, stirring, for 30 seconds, or until the garlic is fragrant but not browned. Add the nomato sauce, then add the chicken and bring the mixture to a simmer. Reduce the heat to low, cover, and cook for 10 to 15 minutes, or until the chicken is firm and cooked through.

Remove from the heat and let cool for 10 minutes, then use your fingers or two forks to shred the chicken.

Chickpea & Kale Curry

VEGAN

Serves 4

This is an old goop detox recipe that I return to again and again. It's easy to throw together, full of flavor, and—bonus—kid-friendly.

3 tablespoons olive oil

1 medium yellow onion

Kosher salt

4 large garlic cloves, minced

3 tablespoons minced fresh ginger

1 teaspoon garam masala

2 teaspoons curry powder

½ teaspoon ground coriander

A small pinch of cayenne pepper

1 (14.5-ounce) can chickpeas, drained and rinsed

1 cup Vegetable Stock (page 192)

1 cup light coconut milk

2 cups packed finely chopped kale leaves (about ½ bunch)

Flaky sea salt

Fresh lemon juice

In a Dutch oven, heat the olive oil over medium heat. Add the onion and a pinch of kosher salt and cook for 7 minutes, or until beginning to soften. Add the garlic, ginger, garam masala, curry powder, coriander, and cayenne and cook for 2 minutes more.

Add the chickpeas, stock, and coconut milk and bring the mixture to a boil. Reduce the heat to maintain a simmer and cook gently for 10 minutes to allow the flavors to meld.

Add the kale and another pinch of salt and simmer gently for 10 minutes more.

Season with flaky salt and pepper and finish with a squeeze of lemon juice just before serving.

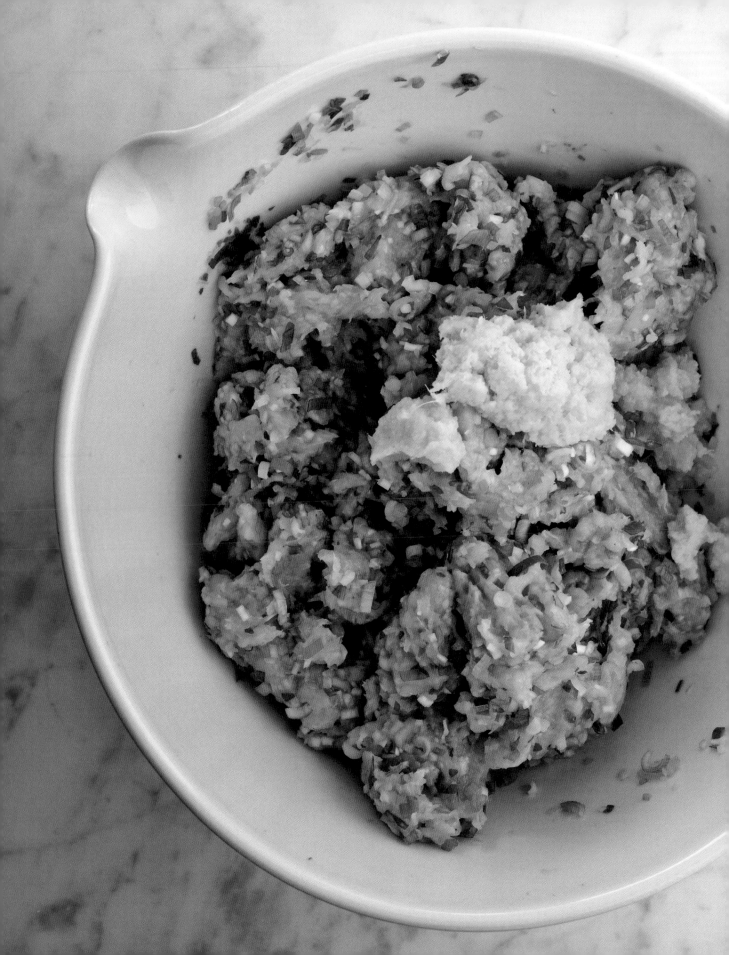

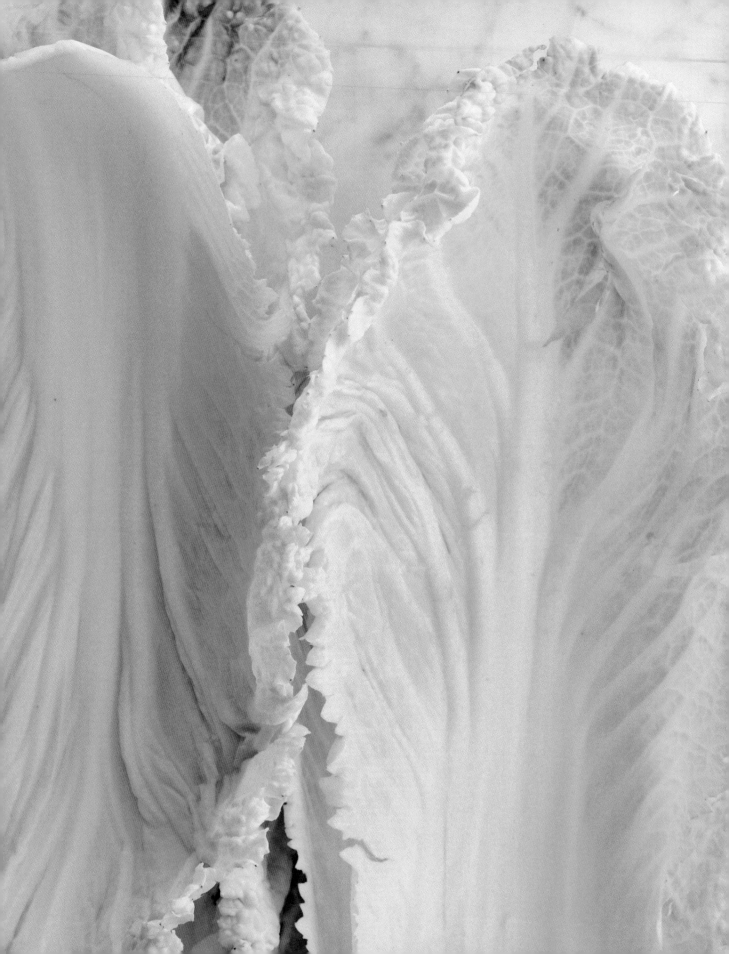

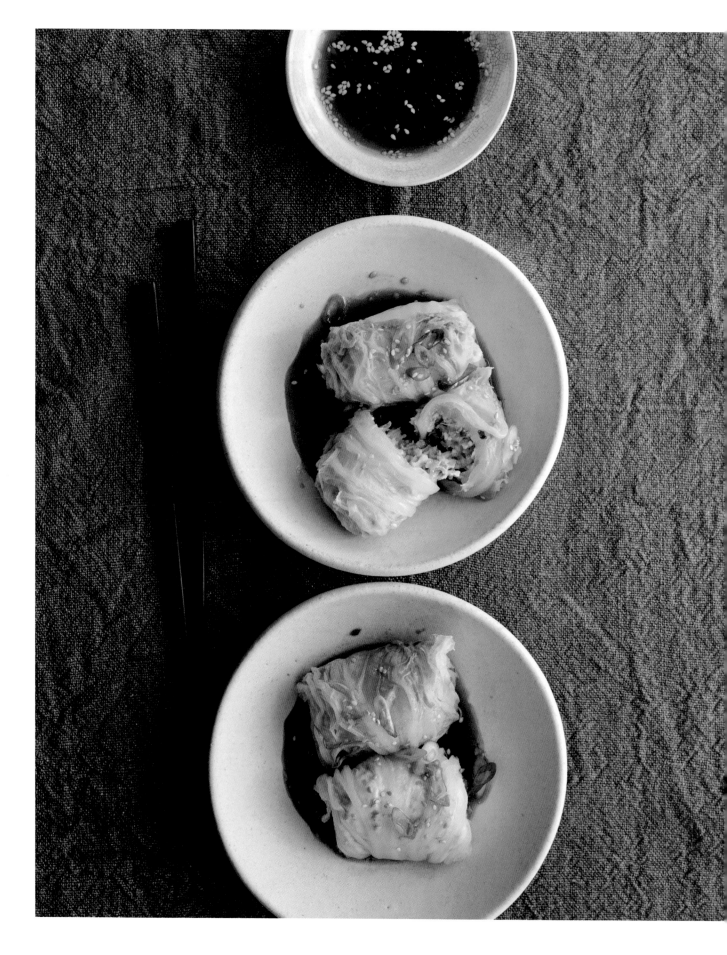

Chicken & Cabbage Dim Sum

Serves 4

This recipe got me through a recent cleanse—turns out, eliminating gluten didn't exactly eliminate my love of dumplings. A sort of dim sum/cabbage roll hybrid, these little parcels are flavorful, satisfying, and fun to make. They're also super versatile—I've made versions with fish or just veggies instead of chicken, and they've all gotten thumbs up.

1 pound dark meat ground chicken

1 bunch of scallions, minced

5 garlic cloves, minced

2 tablespoons minced fresh ginger

1½ teaspoons kosher salt

1 head of green or savoy cabbage

Coconut Aminos Sauce (page 186) for serving

Combine all the ingredients except the cabbage in a large bowl. Mix well, then refrigerate while you prep the cabbage leaves.

Bring a large pot of water to a boil and fill a large bowl with ice and water.

Using a sturdy pair of tongs, place the entire cabbage head into the boiling water and cook for 45 to 60 seconds. Carefully pull the cabbage out. Remove the two or three layers of softened outer leaves and transfer them to the ice bath. Repeat until you have 10 blanched leaves. Dry the leaves well before assembling the rolls.

Place one cabbage leaf on your work surface with the stem end closest to you. Add about 3 tablespoons of the chicken mixture at the base of the cabbage leaf and fold it up and away from you, gently tucking the sides in over your first fold and rolling until you've formed a nice little package. Set aside and repeat to use the remaining cabbage leaves and filling.

Fill a pot with about 1 inch of water and set a wire or bamboo steamer basket inside. Line the bottom of the steamer with any extra blanched cabbage leaves. Bring the water to a simmer.

Set the dumplings in the steamer basket, seam-side down, cover, and steam for about 15 minutes—just until the filling looks cooked and is slightly firm.

Serve with coconut aminos sauce.

Spinach & Pea Curry

<u>QUICK / VEGAN</u>

Serves 2

I was obsessed with the Indian Creamed Spinach from my last cookbook, *It's All Easy*, but I wanted to try to make a vegan version using coconut milk. It's just as creamy and the flavors go so well together. This is the result: a riff on *palak matar*, a spinach and pea curry. It's light and flavorful and works equally well over basmati or cauliflower rice.

1 tablespoon coconut oil

1 garlic clove, grated

1 teaspoon grated fresh ginger

½ teaspoon garam masala

½ teaspoon curry powder

1 cup frozen peas

1 cup full-fat coconut milk

5 ounces baby spinach

Flaky sea salt

In a large sauté pan, melt the coconut oil over medium heat. Add the garlic, ginger, garam masala, and curry powder and cook, stirring occasionally to prevent burning, for a few minutes, until fragrant. Add the peas and coconut milk and cook for about 5 minutes more, gently mashing some of the peas to thicken the mixture. Add the spinach and stir. Simmer for a few more minutes, until the spinach is wilted. Finish with a pinch of flaky salt and serve.

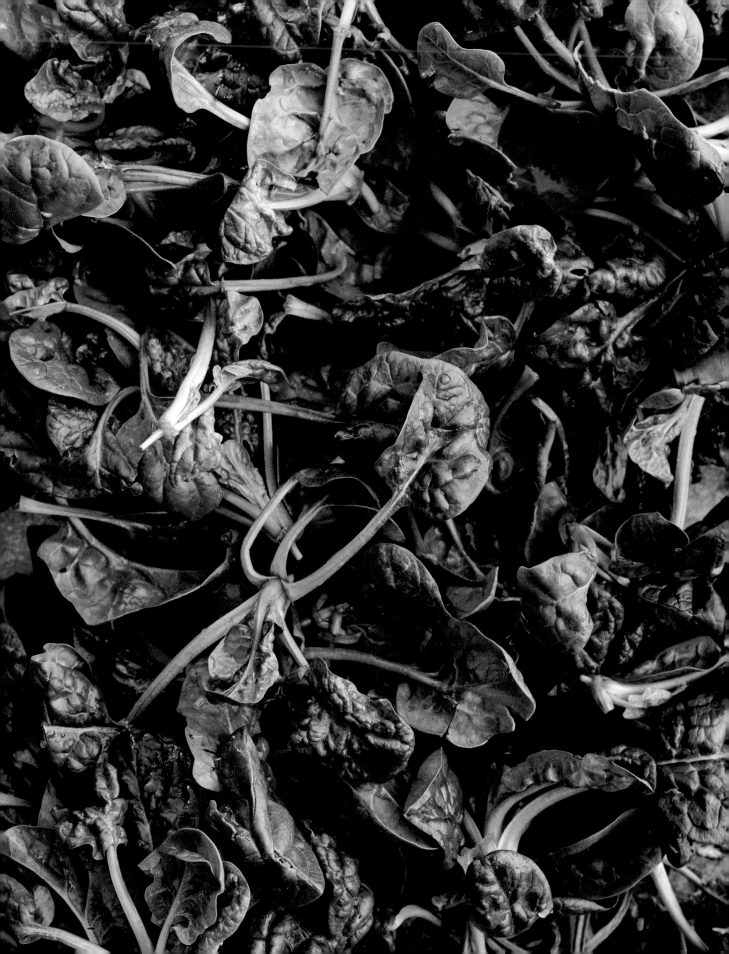

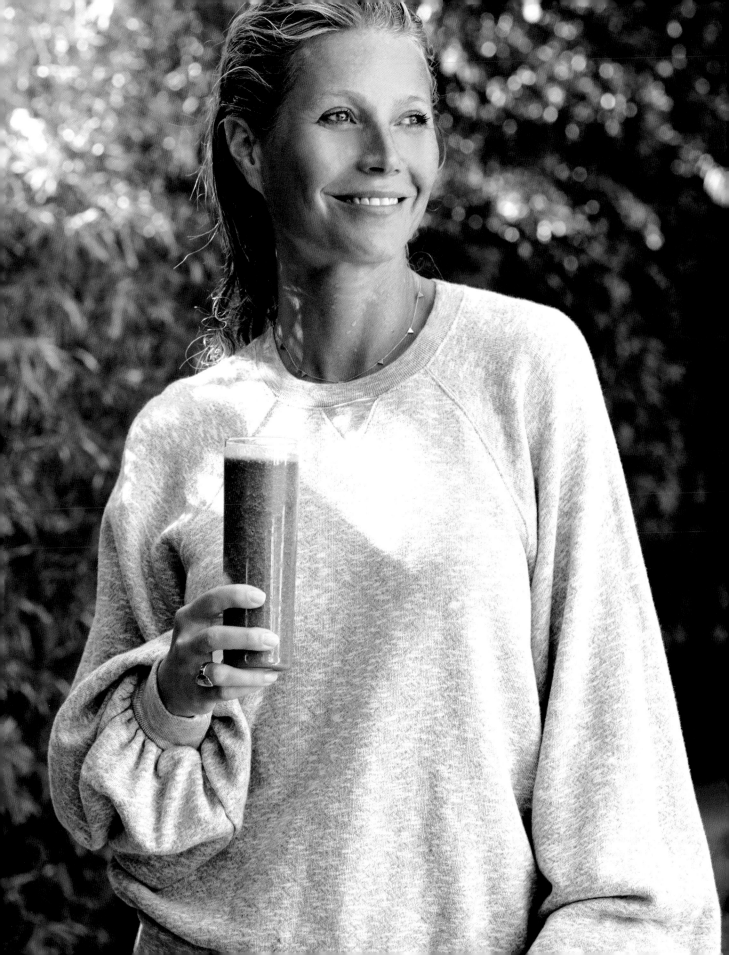

DRINKS & SNACKS

For most people, the hardest part of eating clean isn't breakfast, lunch, or dinner but all the time in between. That eleven a.m. hunger pang or the four p.m. caffeine/sugar craving isn't easy to ignore, particularly when the smell of your work wife's almond milk latte is somehow wafting right over your desk. So instead of depriving myself and simply "pushing through" until the next meal, I rely on an arsenal of delicious snacks and drinks to keep me going—like my dandelion mocha that, while being totally caffeine-free, does a valiant job at scratching a cappuccino itch; cacao date balls that taste as good as a piece of chocolate but have zero refined sugar and give me tons of energy; and a couple of smoothies that do double duty as a breakfast or post-breakfast snack for me, and a post-school snack for my kids.

Cashew Turmeric Iced Latte

<u>VEGAN</u>

Serves 2

This latte is not only pretty, but also packs in hero health ingredient turmeric—extolled by basically every functional practitioner I see—and is naturally caffeine-free. I make a quick cashew milk here, but if you're in a rush or don't have a powerful enough blender on hand, just sub in the same amount of a good (unsweetened) store-bought variety.

1 cup organic raw cashews

1½ cups boiling water

1½ teaspoons ground turmeric

3 dates, pitted

2 cups filtered water

A large pinch of flaky sea salt

Freshly ground black pepper

Place the cashews in a bowl and cover with the boiling water. Let sit for 20 minutes, then drain.

Place the softened cashews in a high-speed blender, add the remaining ingredients, and blend until smooth.

Strain through a fine-mesh sieve or nut milk bag into 2 glasses over ice and serve.

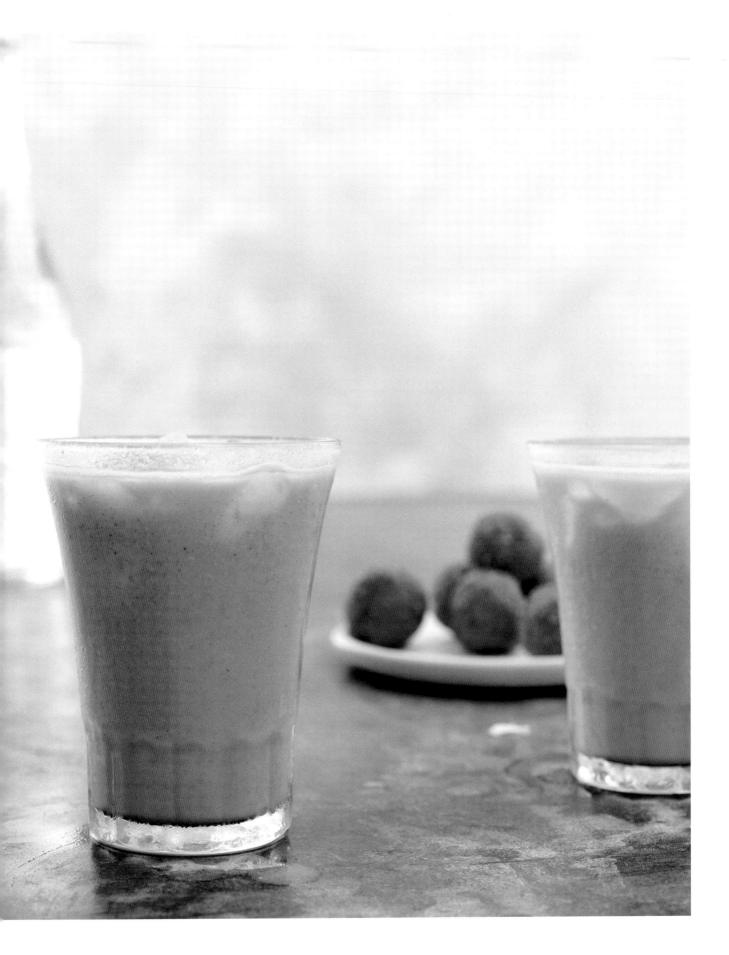

Rosemary Sea Salt Nuts

PACKABLE / QUICK / VEGAN

Makes 1 cup

The hardest part of eliminating processed foods is losing your beloved snacks. Luckily there are plenty of clean snack opportunities. This is one of my faves—delicious and couldn't be easier to pull off. We all deserve a zesty snack, detox or not.

1 cup pecans

2 tablespoons neutral oil (such as grapeseed oil)

Zest and juice of 1 lemon

¼ cup fresh rosemary, chopped

1 teaspoon flaky sea salt

Preheat the oven to 375°F. Line a baking sheet with parchment paper.

Combine all the ingredients in a medium bowl. Spread the nuts over the prepared baking sheet. Bake for 15 to 18 minutes, tossing and turning the nuts a few times as they bake.

As soon as the nuts are done, toss with salt. Let cool completely before serving.

Everything Bagel Cashews

PACKABLE / QUICK / VEGAN

Makes 1 cup

Cashews are one of my favorite midday snacks. They're packable and filling, satisfying that after-lunch craving for something crunchy. But a handful of raw nuts can only get you so far, which is why I wanted to combine them with one of my other favorite but not-so-clean foods: the everything bagel. They're a great way to satisfy that craving without all the schmear.

1 cup raw cashews

1 tablespoon neutral oil (such as sunflower seed oil)

2 teaspoons crushed dried onion

1 teaspoon onion powder

2 teaspoons crushed dried garlic

1 teaspoon garlic powder

1 teaspoon sesame seeds

1 teaspoon poppy seeds

1 teaspoon coarse salt

Preheat the oven to 375°F. Line a baking sheet with parchment paper.

Combine the cashews and oil in a medium bowl. Spread the nuts over the prepared baking sheet. Bake for 15 to 18 minutes, tossing and turning the nuts a few times as they bake.

In another medium bowl, combine the dried onion, onion powder, dried garlic, garlic powder, sesame seeds, poppy seeds, and salt. As soon as the nuts are done, toss with the spice mix. Let them cool before serving.

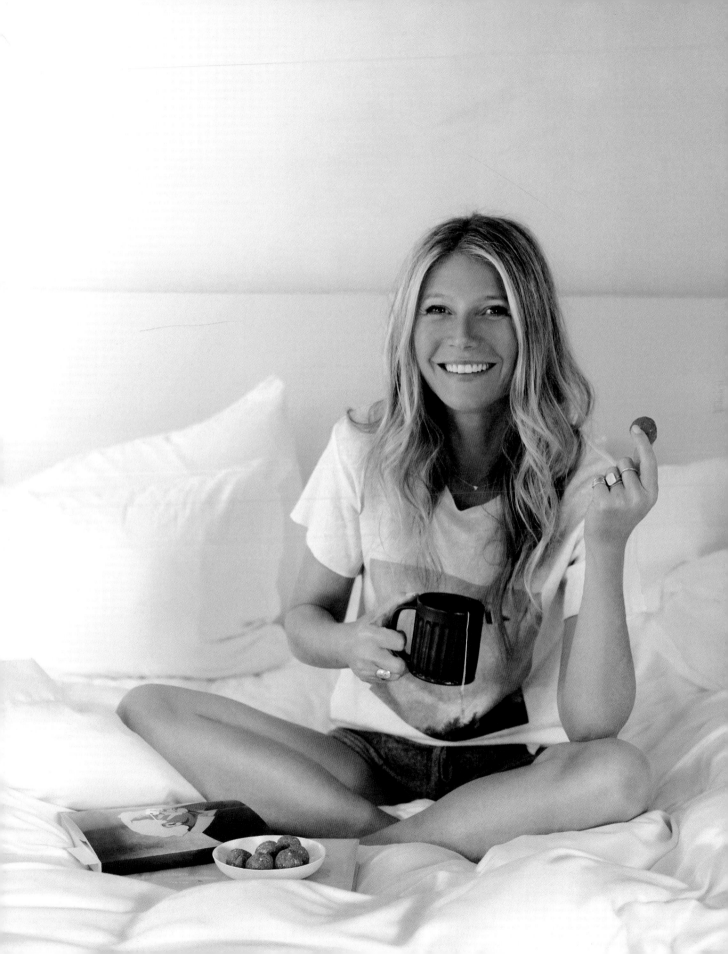

Apricot, Cashew & Coconut Truffles

PACKABLE / QUICK / VEGAN

Makes 12 balls

These fruity, tropical bites are made for an afternoon treat; they're also great for packing in the kids' lunches. Treats all around!

½ **cup dried apricots**

½ **cup raw cashews**

½ **cup unsweetened shredded coconut**

Zest of 1 lime

A pinch of flaky sea salt

1 tablespoon water

Combine all the ingredients in a food processor and process until the mixture is smooth and forms a ball around the processor blade (this may take a while).

Using wet hands, roll the mixture into 12 tablespoon-sized balls, setting them on a plate as you work.

Let set in the fridge until ready to eat.

Mango Lassi

PACKABLE / QUICK / VEGAN

Serves 1

A play on a mango lassi, this refreshing drink uses coconut milk in place of yogurt and gets a color boost from a little ground turmeric.

½ cup coconut water

½ cup fresh mango

¼ teaspoon ground turmeric

¼ cup unsweetened full-fat coconut milk

A pinch of flaky sea salt

Combine all the ingredients in a high-speed blender and blend until smooth.

Pour into a glass over ice and serve.

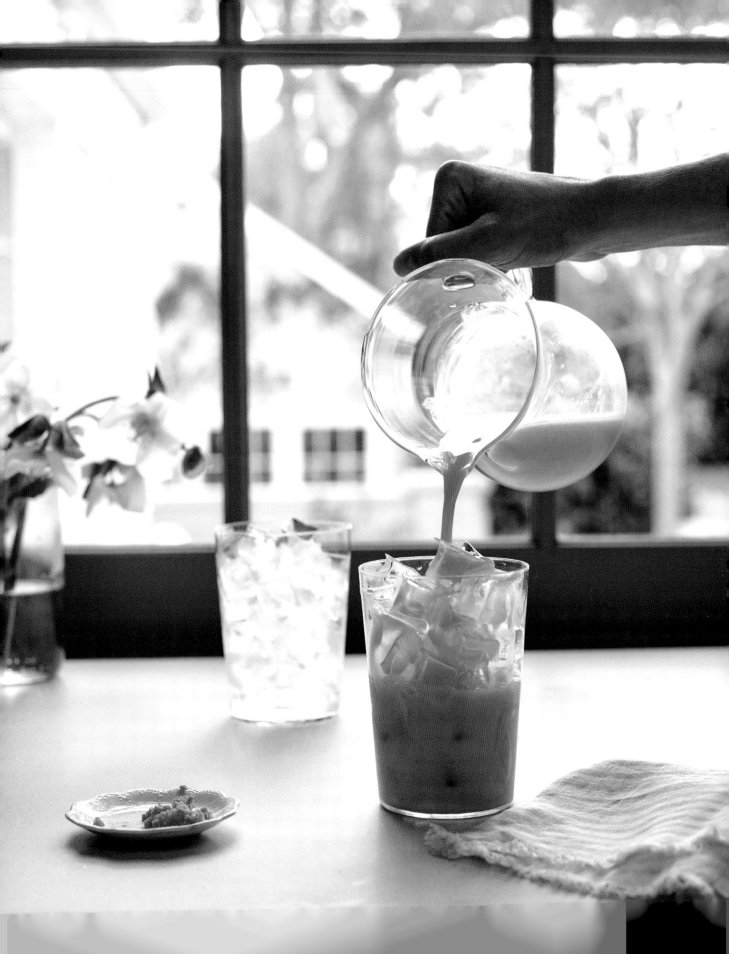

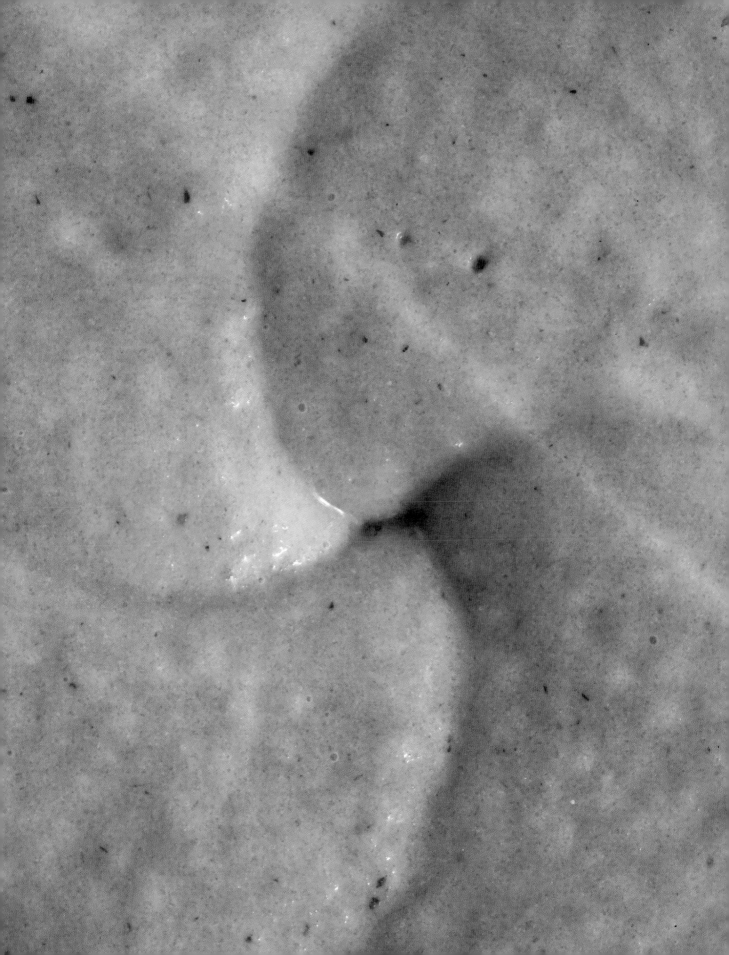

Strawberry Cauliflower Smoothie

PACKABLE / QUICK / VEGAN

Serves 1

I know, I know, frozen cauliflower in a smoothie sounds gross, but it adds incredible creaminess without all the sugar of bananas (on the "no" list for set cleanses like Dr. Junger's Clean Program) and, paired with tropical fruit and lime, actually tastes really good. Even my kids happily slurp it down for breakfast or an afternoon snack. If you're sensitive to strawberries, try pineapple here instead.

½ cup frozen cauliflower

½ cup frozen mango

½ cup frozen strawberries (optional)

½ cup coconut water

2 tablespoons unsweetened canned or refrigerated coconut milk

Juice of ½ lime

Combine all the ingredients in a high-speed blender and blend until smooth.

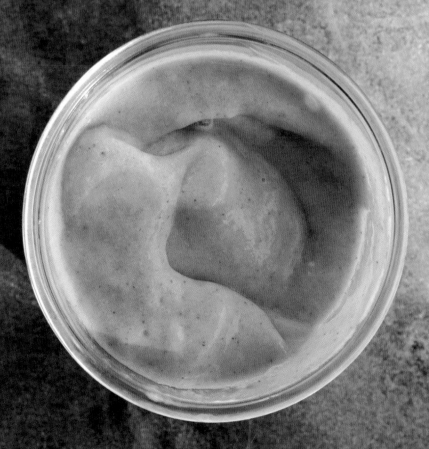

Blueberry Cauliflower Smoothie

PACKABLE / QUICK / VEGAN

Serves 1

With antioxidant-rich blueberries and protein-packed almond butter, this smoothie is one I often throw together after a workout. Buy organic wild blueberries, if you can find them.

½ cup frozen blueberries
½ cup frozen cauliflower
1 tablespoon unsweetened almond butter
¾ cup unsweetened almond milk
1 date, pitted and roughly chopped
Juice of ½ lime

Combine all the ingredients in a high-speed blender and blend until smooth.

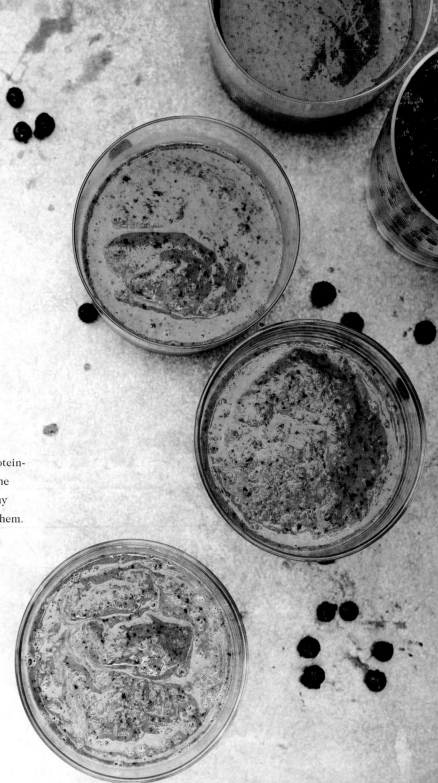

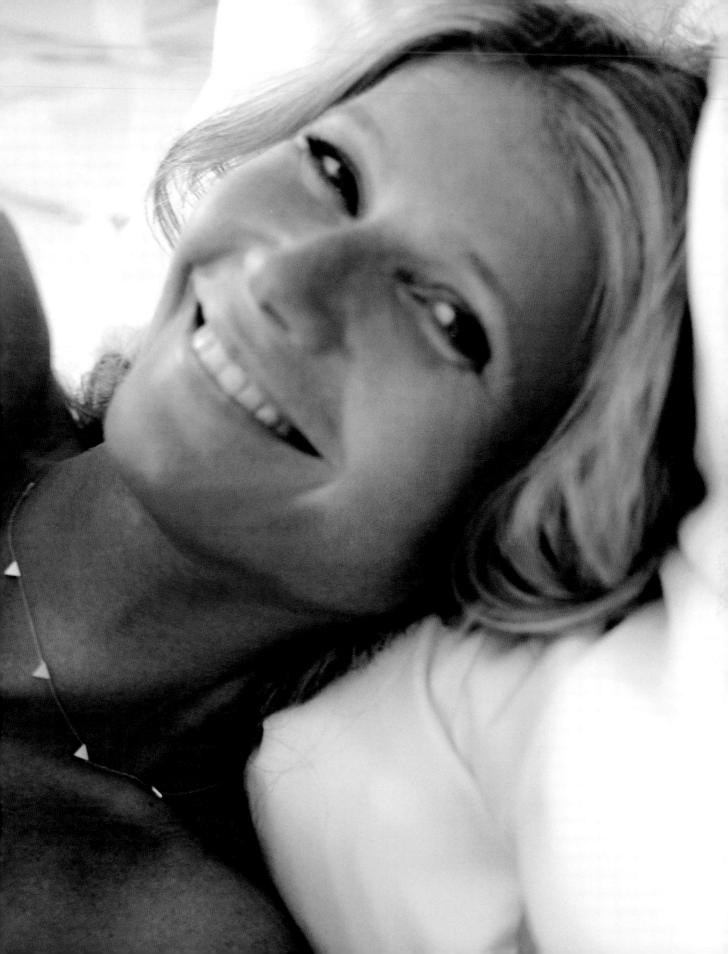

Chlorella Smoothie

PACKABLE / QUICK / VEGAN

Serves 1

A freshwater algae that happens to be a complete
plant protein, chlorella is also thought to be a
good chelator (see more on chelation from
Dr. Novak on page 227). I pair it with fruit and
fresh mint to balance its slightly mossy flavor.

¼ cup frozen mango

¼ cup frozen peach

½ cup spinach

¼ cup full-fat coconut milk

½ teaspoon monk fruit or liquid stevia (not stevia-
based sweetener)

¼ teaspoon chlorella

6 fresh mint leaves

Combine all the ingredients in a high-speed blender
and blend until creamy and smooth.

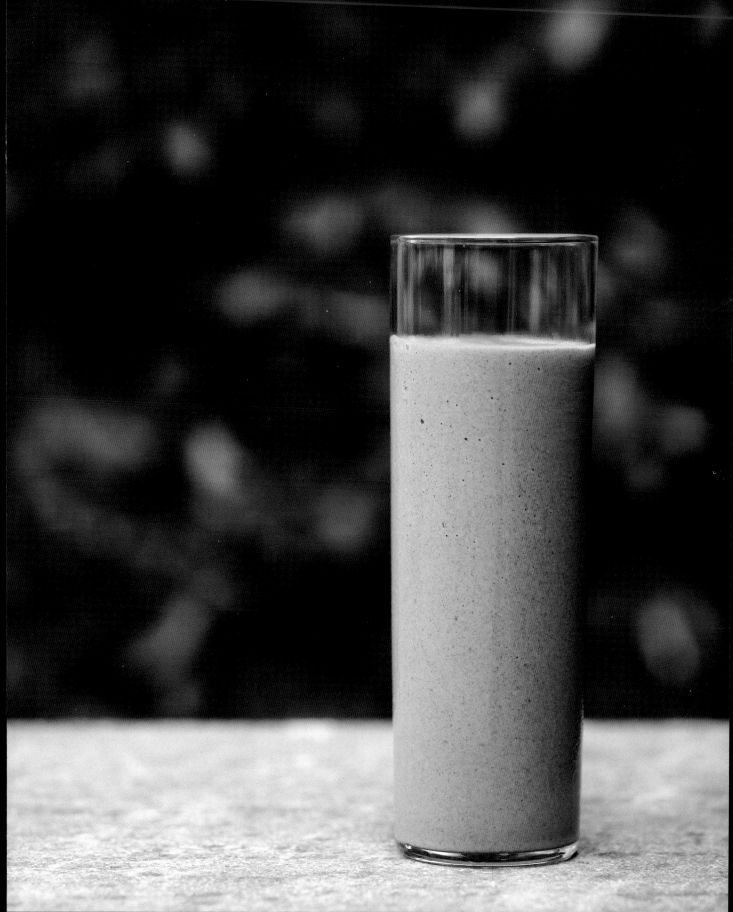

Cacao Date Truffles

PACKABLE / QUICK / VEGAN

Makes 12 balls

I'm not a big dessert person (I know, I know, what's wrong with me?), but every once in a while I crave something sweet and chocolatey, and these cacao date balls really hit the spot. Plus, there's the added bonus of satisfying your chocolate craving with iron- and antioxidant-rich raw cacao (which I've been told is good for the heart—see page 248). Ashwagandha is an adaptogenic herb that may help with stress, so you can add that also if you'd like (you can find both raw cacao and ashwagandha in health food stores or online). Make a double batch and store them in the fridge to combat candy bar cravings at any time.

½ cup pitted Medjool dates

½ cup raw cashews

½ cup raw almonds, preferably sprouted

⅛ teaspoon vanilla powder

¼ teaspoon ashwagandha (optional)

1 tablespoon raw cacao powder

A large pinch of flaky sea salt

2 tablespoons water

2 tablespoons cacao nibs

Combine the dates, cashews, almonds, vanilla, ashwagandha (if using), cacao, salt, and water in a food processor and process until the mixture is smooth and forms a ball. Mix in the cacao nibs by hand.

Using wet hands, shape the mixture into 12 tablespoon-sized balls, setting them on a plate as you work.

Store in the fridge until ready to eat.

Ginger & Cilantro Tea

Serves 2

Cilantro is thought to have great detoxifying properties, and adding it to a tea is an easy way to get a dose. The addition of ginger to this tea makes it so soothing that you'll want to make it part of your everyday routine.

2½ cups water

1 (2-inch) piece fresh ginger, cut in half lengthwise

4 cilantro sprigs

In a small saucepan, bring the water to a boil. Add the ginger and cilantro, reduce the heat to low, and simmer for 3 to 4 minutes.

Strain into 2 mugs and discard the ginger and cilantro. Enjoy.

Chamomile & Mint Tea

Serves 1

Reducing stress and getting enough rest are essential to overall wellness. This tea is an easy (and tasty) way to help you wind down after a hectic day. Ethereal and light chamomile paired with fresh, cleansing mint make for a delightfully warm cuppa.

2½ cups water

1 tablespoon dried chamomile

1 tablespoon dried mint leaves

In a small saucepan, bring the water to a boil. Combine the chamomile and mint in a teabag or infuser and place it in a mug. Pour over the boiling water and steep for 3 to 6 minutes, depending on how strong you prefer your tea.

Remove the teabag or infuser and enjoy.

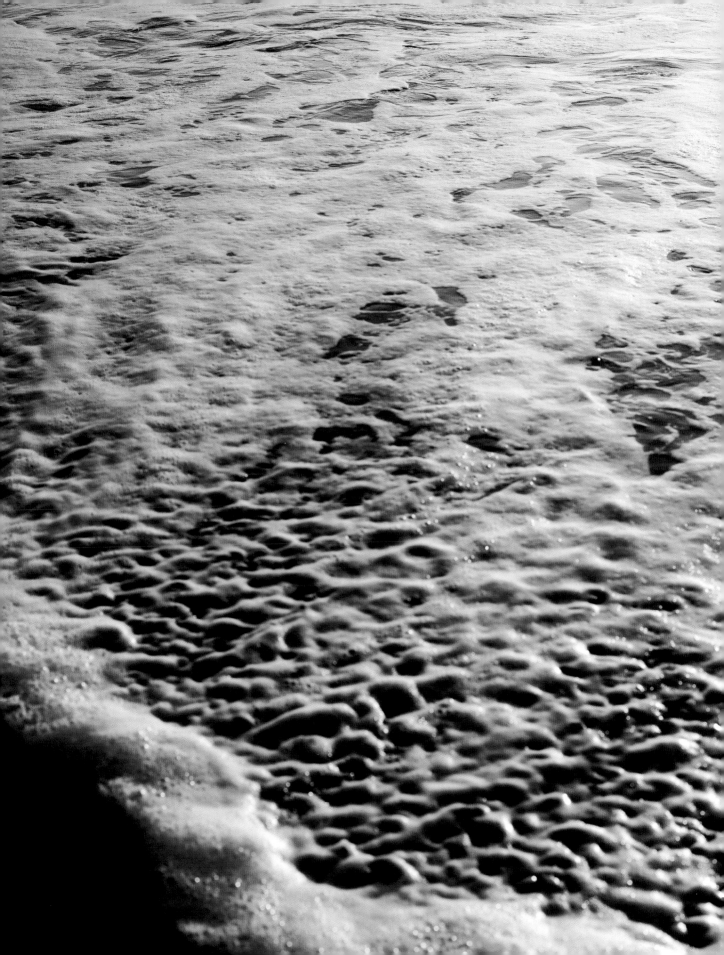

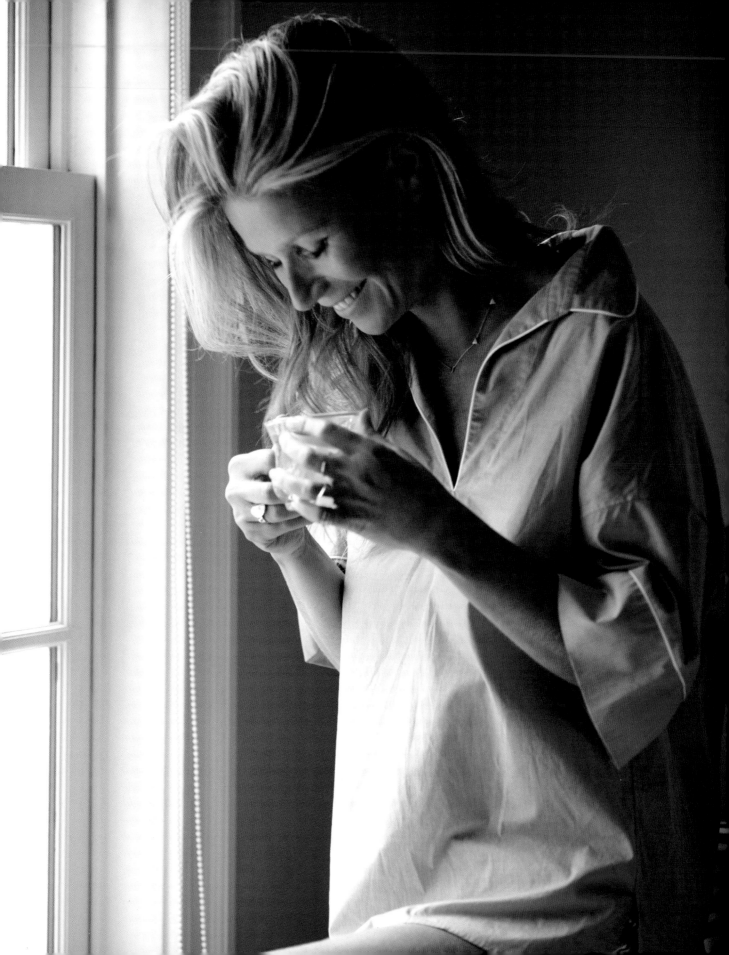

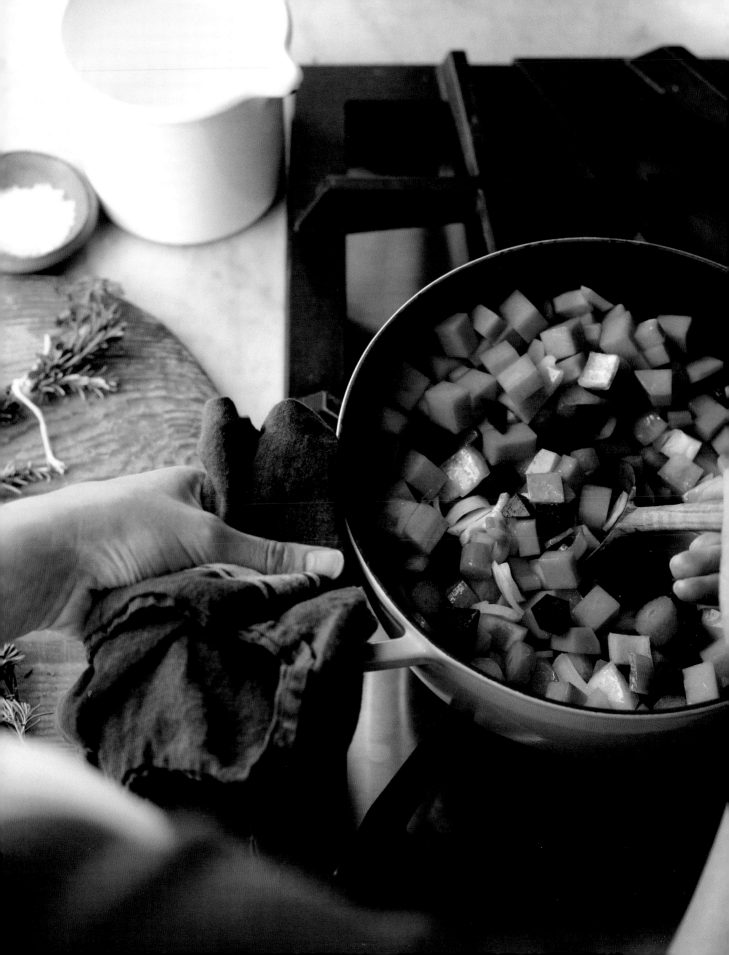

BASICS

While the basics section of any cookbook is important, it's arguably *especially* crucial here, because the majority of store-bought sauces, condiments, and snacks are no-go's on a full-out clean-eating plan (they tend to be full of hidden additives, gluten, and sugar). This chapter is full of super-flavorful clean versions of my fridge and pantry staples, including delicious sugar- and vinegar-free salad dressings; a soy-free dipping sauce that's perfect for hand rolls, salads, and grain bowls; a tomato-free sauce that both looks and tastes remarkably like marinara; and a magical vegan mayonnaise made from the liquid from a can of chickpeas (I'm serious). Yes, cooking from scratch like this takes a little time, but once you're stocked up with a few of these basics, the recipes in the other chapters will come together quickly and easily. Plus, with this repertoire of clean-eating building blocks under your belt, you'll be able to adapt and improvise, whipping up, say, a clean nomato lasagna or drizzling a dressing over a perfect grain bowl. Once you've got the basics down, the possibilities are endless.

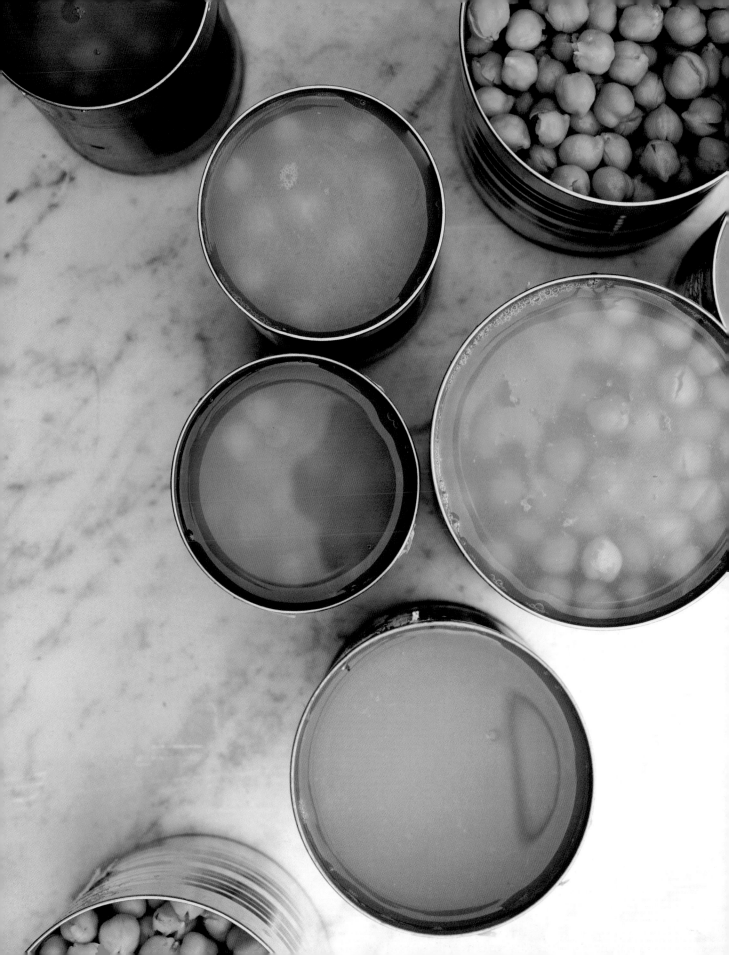

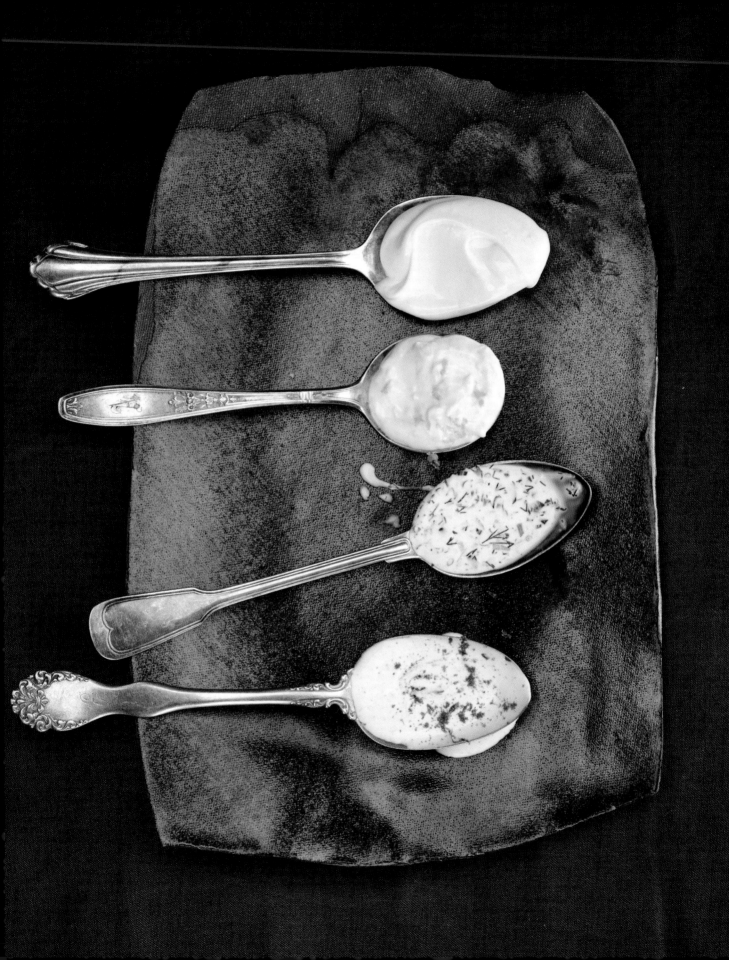

Aquafaba Mayo

Makes about 2 cups

Aquafaba mayo is a clean-eating game changer. For the homemade egg-free mayo of your dreams, you emulsify aquafaba—the liquid from a can of chickpeas—with a neutral oil for several minutes. The best part is that it makes an ideal neutral base for any flavored aioli you can think of. I came up with three tasty riffs, but that's just to get you started. Try swirling in some vegan pesto or Tunisian harissa paste (found in most gourmet markets and online) or even Paleo sriracha.

½ cup aquafaba (liquid from a can of organic chickpeas)

1 teaspoon fresh lemon juice

¾ teaspoon kosher salt

About 1½ cups neutral oil (such as sunflower seed or grapeseed oil)

Combine the aquafaba, lemon juice, and salt in a small bowl. Using an immersion blender on a medium-high speed, pour in the oil in a very slow, steady stream. The aquafaba should begin to stiffen and expand—this will take a few minutes; it will be smooth and thickened.

Transfer the mayo to an airtight container and store in the fridge for up to about a week.

Lemony Garlic Aquafaba Sauce

QUICK / VEGAN

Makes about ½ cup

This egg-free sauce is great when you're missing that creamy "special sauce" on your burger. But beyond that, use it with abandon—it plays well with wraps or works dolloped on a grain bowl, and I especially love it as a dip for roasted sweet potato wedges.

½ cup Aquafaba Mayo (page 178)

1 garlic clove, grated

Zest of ½ lemon

½ teaspoon fresh lemon juice

Combine all the ingredients in a small bowl and gently mix. Cover and store in a jar with a lid in the fridge for up to 1 week.

Aquafaba Crema

QUICK / VEGAN

Makes about ½ cup

There's no real replacement for sour cream on a taco, but this comes pretty close. It's creamy and citrusy, and the earthy, savory flavor of cumin will make you forget it's vegan (no small feat).

½ cup Aquafaba Mayo (page 178)

¼ teaspoon ground cumin

Juice of ½ lime

Kosher salt

Combine all the ingredients in a small bowl and gently mix. Cover and store in a jar with a lid in the fridge for up to 1 week.

Aquafaba Ranch Dressing

QUICK / VEGAN

Makes about ½ cup

You'll have a hard time going back to old-school ranch dressing once you try this. It's incredibly flavorful and packed full of fresh herbs, and not full of dairy and gluten—not to mention the additives and preservatives listed on the back of store bottles that I can't even pronounce. Serve it with crudités, or in the crunchy garden salad on page 59.

½ cup Aquafaba Mayo (page 178)

Zest and juice of ½ lemon

1 garlic clove, grated

1 shallot, minced

1 teaspoon finely chopped fresh dill

1 tablespoon finely chopped fresh parsley

1 tablespoon finely chopped fresh chives

¼ teaspoon kosher salt

¼ teaspoon freshly ground black pepper

Combine all the ingredients in a small bowl and gently mix. Cover and store in a jar with a lid in the fridge for up to 1 week.

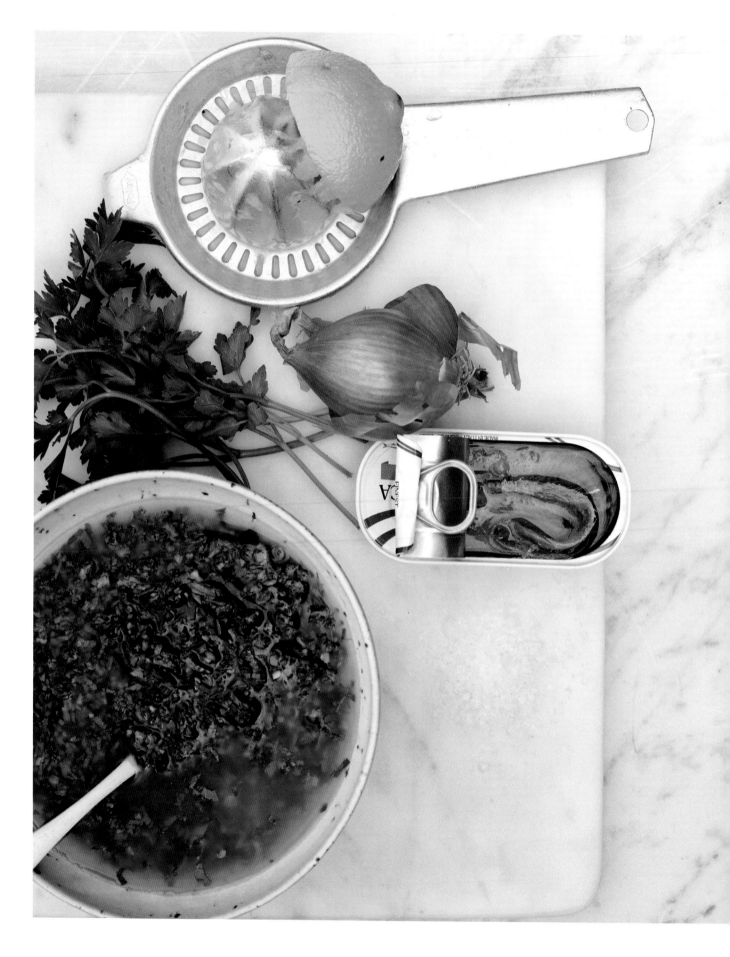

Parsley Salsa Verde

QUICK

Makes about ⅔ cup

This is one of my all-time favorite condiments. The briny flavor of anchovies, with bright parsley and a little bite from raw shallot is just beyond. You can pretty much vary it however you like—try adding garlic, capers, or even thyme to the mix.

1 bunch of parsley, chopped

1 tablespoon shallot, finely chopped

½ teaspoon grated lemon zest

¼ teaspoon kosher salt

¼ teaspoon chili flakes (optional)

4 anchovy fillets, chopped (optional)

⅔ cup extra virgin olive oil

Combine all the ingredients in a small bowl and mix well to combine. Cover and store in the fridge for up to 1 week.

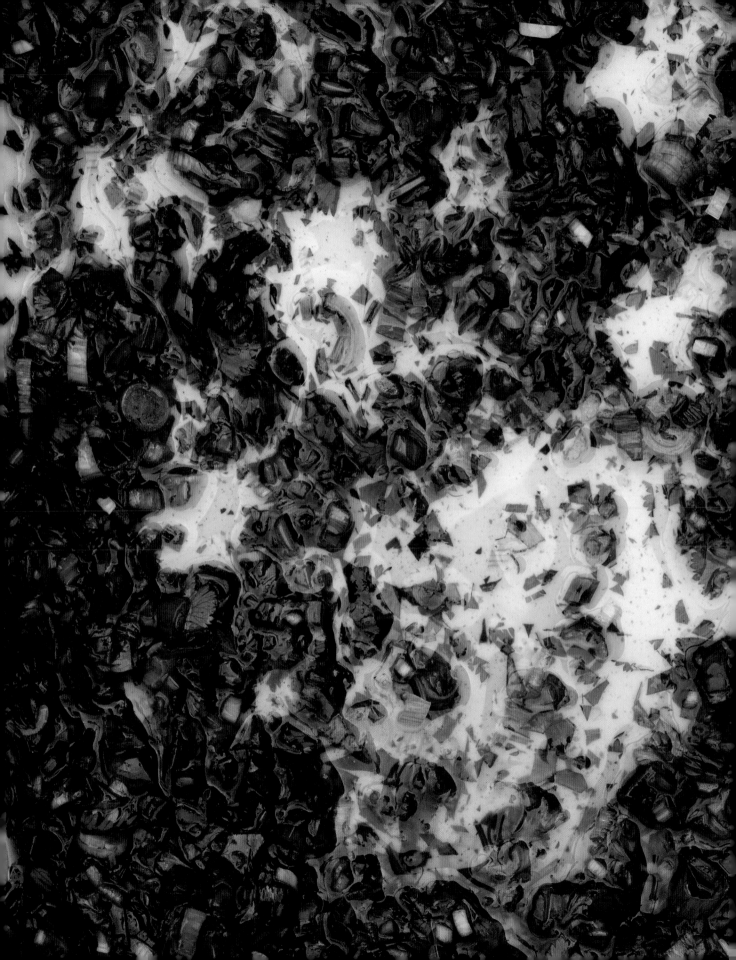

Cilantro Salsa Verde

QUICK / VEGAN

Makes about ⅔ cup

A light, herby salsa verde can brighten up everything from soups to grilled fish to poached eggs. This one is a little different, as it uses cilantro, lime, and cumin, giving it some earthy flavors to balance the citrus notes.

1 bunch of cilantro, chopped

4 scallions, finely chopped

Zest of ½ lime

¼ teaspoon ground cumin

¼ teaspoon kosher salt

⅔ cup extra virgin olive oil

Combine all the ingredients in a small bowl and mix well. Cover and store in the fridge for up to 1 week.

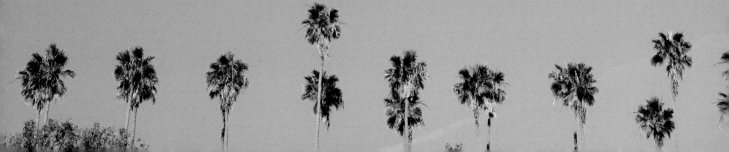

Coconut Aminos Sauce

QUICK / VEGAN

Makes about ⅓ cup

A soy-free version of my go-to dipping sauce is a reality thanks to coconut aminos, aka fermented coconut nectar, whose natural sweetness lends an almost teriyaki flavor to any dish it's used in. It's the bomb. And this easy condiment is sure to become your go-to for an extra pop of flavor on dumplings, hand rolls, and cauli bowls.

¼ cup coconut aminos

Juice of 1 lime

½ teaspoon grated fresh ginger

1 tablespoon toasted sesame oil

½ teaspoon sesame seeds

Combine all the ingredients in a small bowl and whisk together.

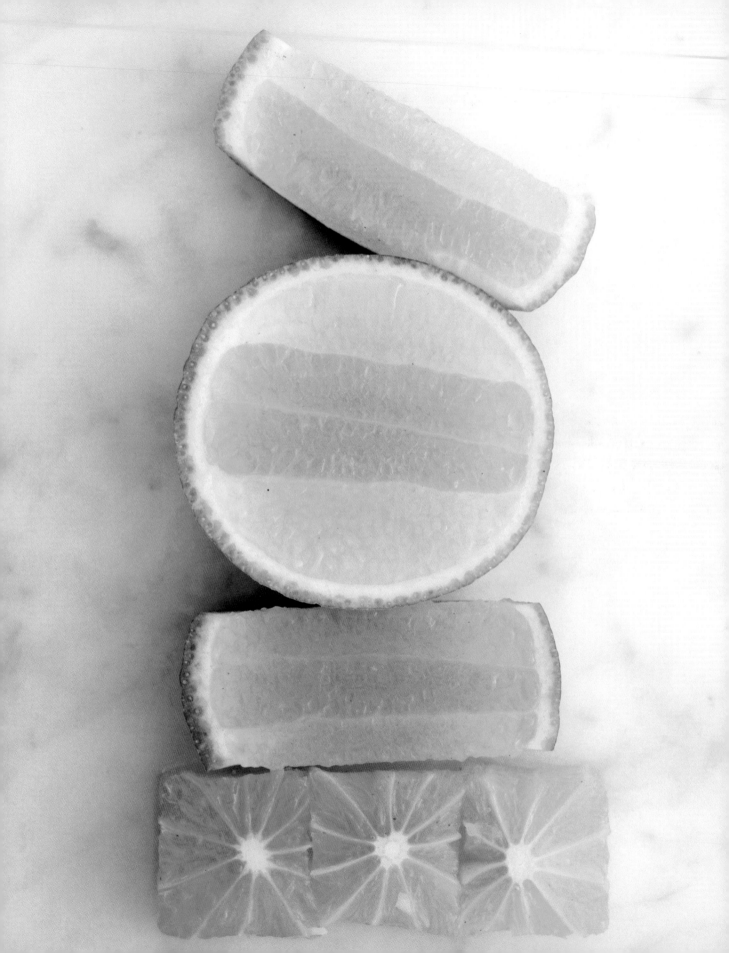

Miso-Ginger Dressing

QUICK / VEGAN

Makes about ½ cup

Miso is one of my favorite ingredients. Switching to chickpea miso—which is made by fermenting chickpeas instead of soybeans—allows me to enjoy it even when I'm eating clean. You can find chickpea miso in most health food stores and online.

2 teaspoons chickpea miso paste

2 teaspoons grated fresh ginger

Zest and juice of 2 limes

½ cup extra virgin olive oil

Flaky sea salt

In a small bowl, whisk together the miso, ginger, lime zest, and lime juice. While whisking continuously, slowly add the olive oil, then whisk until emulsified. Taste and season with salt. Cover and store in the fridge for up to 1 week.

Tahini Dressing

QUICK / VEGAN

Makes about ½ cup

Tahini can easily overpower a recipe, but it's one of the best vegan alternatives for creamy dressings. Thinned out with water and balanced with super-savory garlic and shallots, this dressing has the potential to become your new everything sauce.

¼ cup tahini

¼ cup water

2 garlic cloves, grated

Juice of ½ lemon

1 tablespoon apple cider vinegar

2 small shallots, minced

¼ teaspoon kosher salt

In a small bowl, whisk the tahini briefly to loosen it. While whisking continuously, slowly stream in the water; the mixture might seize up and be quite thick, but keep whisking and adding the water until it smooths out (it'll take a minute). Once it has smoothed out and become a bit looser, whisk in the garlic, lemon juice, vinegar, shallots, and salt until combined. Cover and store in the fridge for up to 1 week.

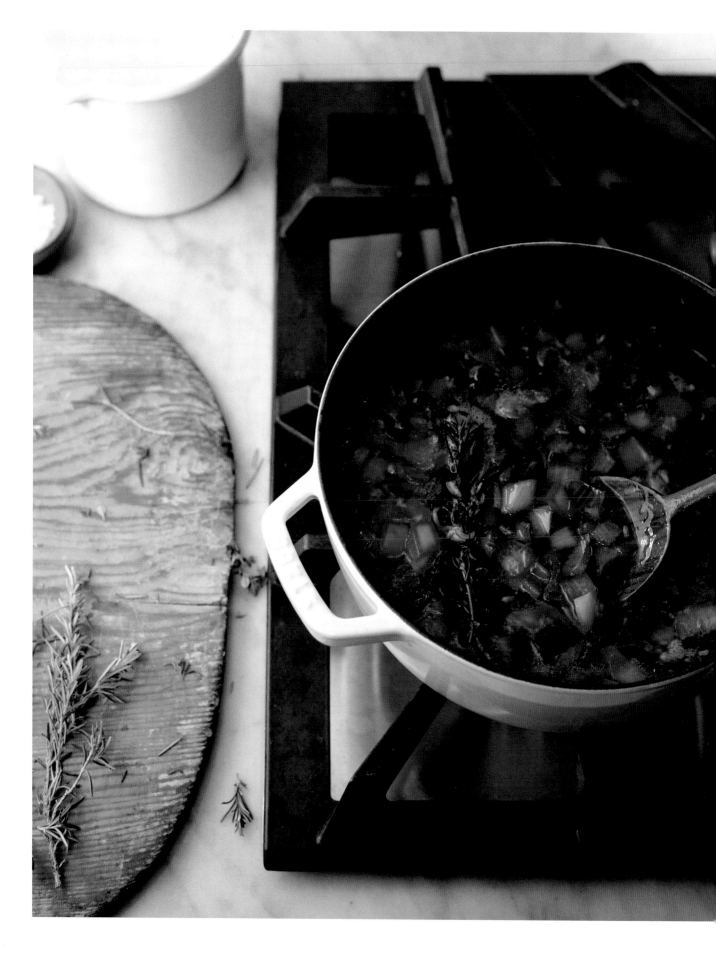

Nomato Sauce

Makes about 6 cups

Eliminating nightshades—vegetables in the Solanaceae family, like tomatoes, peppers, and eggplant, which may trigger inflammation in some people—can be tricky; those flavors and textures are not easy to replace. I found that butternut squash and beets could mimic the texture and color of tomato sauce, and that by pairing the "nomato" sauce with foods and aromatics you'd normally eat with tomato sauce (herbs, fennel, meatballs, etc.), you don't really miss the actual tomatoes. It's a good solution for a hearty, comforting meal that still plays by super-clean rules.

3 tablespoons olive oil

1 large yellow onion, chopped (about 2½ cups)

3 celery stalks, chopped (about 1½ cups)

6 small carrots, chopped (about 1 cup)

½ small butternut squash, peeled, seeded, and chopped (about 2 cups)

1 small beet, peeled and chopped (about 1 cup)

4 garlic cloves

¼ teaspoon fennel seeds

Bouquet garni: 2 thyme sprigs, 2 rosemary sprigs, and 2 bay leaves, tied together with kitchen twine

1 tablespoon kosher salt

¼ teaspoon freshly ground black pepper

4 cups water

In a large, heavy-bottomed saucepan, heat the olive oil over medium heat. Add the onion, celery, carrot, squash, beet, and garlic and cook, stirring, for about 5 minutes. Add the fennel seeds, bouquet garni, salt, and pepper and cook for 5 minutes or so more. Add the water, reduce the heat to medium-low, partially cover the pot, and cook for about 45 minutes, or until all the vegetables are soft. Discard the bouquet garni and let the sauce cool. Carefully transfer the mixture to a high-speed blender and blend until smooth. (Work in batches, if necessary, and be careful when blending hot or still-warm liquids.)

If the sauce is thinner than you like, return it to the pot and simmer over medium-high heat for about 10 minutes, until thickened and reduced to your liking.

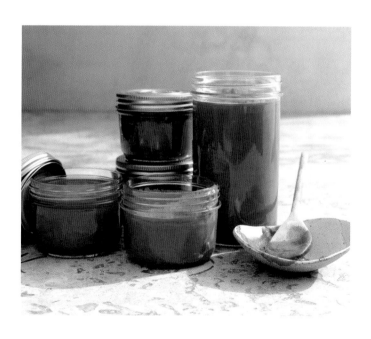

Vegetable Stock

<u>VEGAN</u>

Makes about 8 cups

I'm not a big fan of boxed or canned vegetable stock, especially when it's so easy to make at home. You essentially throw everything in water and let it do its thing. This is a great recipe to store in the freezer for last-minute dinners. I like to buy everything from the farmers' market—that way, I get the brightest, freshest flavors in the stock.

3 tablespoons olive oil

1 red onion, cut in half

1 yellow onion, cut in half

1 bunch of celery, cut into thirds

1 large parsnip, cut in half

1 large carrot, cut in half

1 head of garlic, cut in half

10 cups water

1 teaspoon kosher salt

1 teaspoon whole black peppercorns

1 bay leaf

8 parsley sprigs

In a large stockpot, heat the olive oil over medium-high heat. Add the onions, celery, parsnip, carrot, and garlic. Cook, stirring often, for 5 to 8 minutes, until vegetables become aromatic and soften slightly.

Add the water and stir. Add the salt, peppercorns, bay leaf, and parsley. Bring to a boil, then reduce the heat to maintain a simmer. Cover the pot and simmer for 1½ hours.

Carefully strain the stock and discard the solids. Use immediately or let cool completely, then store in airtight containers in the fridge for up to 1 week or in the freezer for up to 3 months.

Chicken Stock

Makes about 6 cups

Boxed and canned chicken stocks are not my favorite, so when I have the time, I make a batch of my own. I like to use chicken feet, which contain beneficial collagen—great for the gut and joints—but if you can't find them (or if they freak you out), you can absolutely skip them. Ideally, though, you want whatever chicken pieces you're using to be organic and pasture-raised.

2 fresh or frozen chicken carcasses (about 1 pound)

½ pound chicken feet (optional)

1 medium carrot, cut in half

1 large celery stalk, cut in half

1 medium leek, washed well and cut in half

2 teaspoons whole black peppercorns

1 bay leaf

8 cups water

Place the chicken pieces, chicken feet (if using), carrot, celery, leek, peppercorns, and bay leaf in a very large Dutch oven or stockpot. Add the water and bring to a simmer over medium heat. Skim off any scum from the surface with a ladle, then reduce the heat to maintain a very gentle simmer and cook for 1 hour, skimming the surface every 20 minutes or so.

Fill a large bowl with ice and set a second large bowl on top. Strain the stock into the large bowl, discard the solids, and let cool.

Transfer the stock to airtight containers and store in the fridge for up to 1 week or in the freezer for up to 1 month.

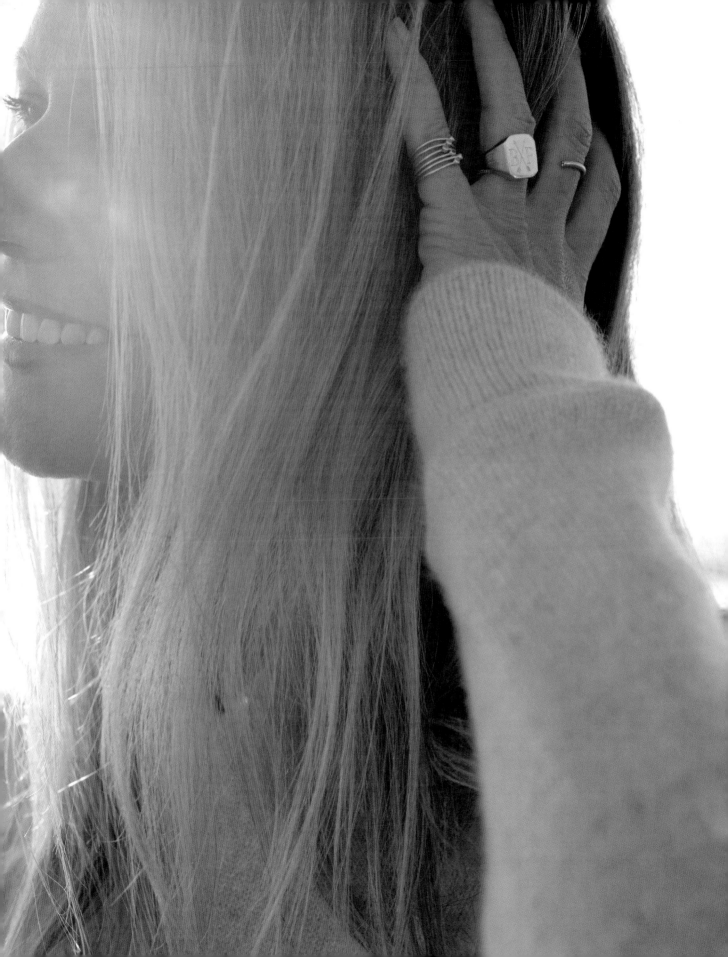

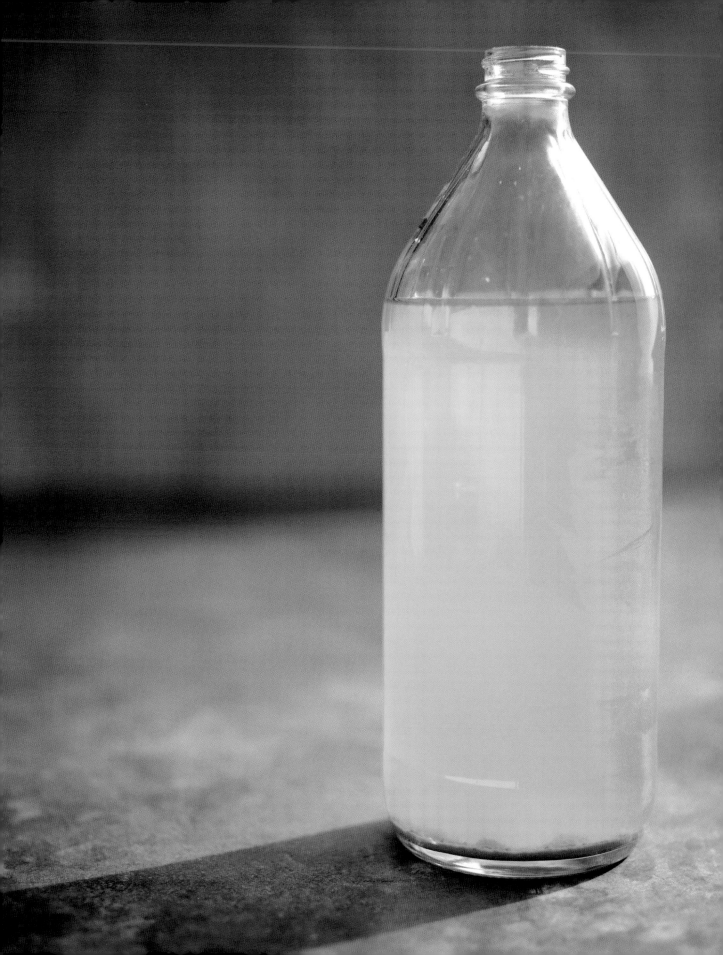

Poached Chicken

Makes 2 chicken breasts

A solid poached chicken breast is a staple in any cook's arsenal, and is particularly handy in a clean-leaning cook's arsenal. It doesn't get much cleaner than water and herbs! You can use poached chicken in just about anything—toss it in a cauliflower rice bowl or a lettuce cup, on a salad, or in a soup. This is the basic recipe, but feel free to add different aromatics to change up the flavor—celery, carrots, parsley, cilantro, garlic, ginger, and lemongrass are just a few ideas.

1 white onion, quartered

½ teaspoon whole black peppercorns

½ teaspoon kosher salt

2 boneless, skinless chicken breasts

In a small saucepan, combine all the ingredients. Add just enough water to cover the chicken. Bring to a boil, then reduce the heat to medium-low and simmer for 20 to 25 minutes; the chicken should look opaque and (obviously) be cooked through.

Roasted Chicken

Serves 4

I use chicken a fair amount in this book, and while a quick poached chicken breast (page 196) is handy, I also wanted to include a really tasty, simple, and clean roasted chicken recipe. After years of slathering birds with brines and butter and herbs, I finally realized that all you really need is a good-quality organic or pasture-raised chicken and some salt. Since I love the crispy skin, I avoid basting or rubbing oil on the outside—there's enough naturally occurring fat in the bird that will render beautifully, resulting in a perfect roasted chicken.

1 (3- to 4-pound) organic chicken

Heaping 1 tablespoon kosher salt

Preheat the oven to 425°F. Line a rimmed baking sheet with parchment paper and set a wire rack on top.

Set the chicken on the rack. Pat it dry all over with paper towels and sprinkle the salt all over the bird. Roast for 1 to 1½ hours, until an instant-read thermometer registers 165°F. Let rest for 20 minutes before carving.

Roasted Beets in Parchment

<u>VEGAN</u>

Makes 6 beets

I use cooked beets a lot when I'm on a clean-eating kick—their sweet, earthy flavor works well in so many dishes, and they feel heartier than a lot of other veggies. I like to roast them *en papillote*, as cooking with aluminum foil is something I try to avoid, and aluminum is at the top of the list of things to eliminate whenever I've talked with functional doctors about their heavy metal detox protocols (see page 225). Make a batch of these at the beginning of the week and use for everything from tacos (page 100) to gazpacho (page 36) to a quinoa sweet potato grain bowl (page 68).

6 beets, scrubbed

2 tablespoons olive oil

3 tablespoons water

½ teaspoon kosher salt

½ teaspoon cracked black pepper

Preheat the oven to 400°F.

Rub each beet with a bit of the olive oil and place them on one half of a 15×12-inch sheet of parchment paper. Add the water. Sprinkle the beets with the salt and pepper.

Carefully fold the top half of the parchment paper over the beets. Starting with one side, roll and crimp the edges of the parchment, making sure no liquid can escape and the beets are completely enclosed. Repeat with the remaining two sides.

Place the parcel on a rimmed baking sheet and roast for 90 minutes.

Remove from the oven, carefully open the parchment (the steam inside is hot), and serve.

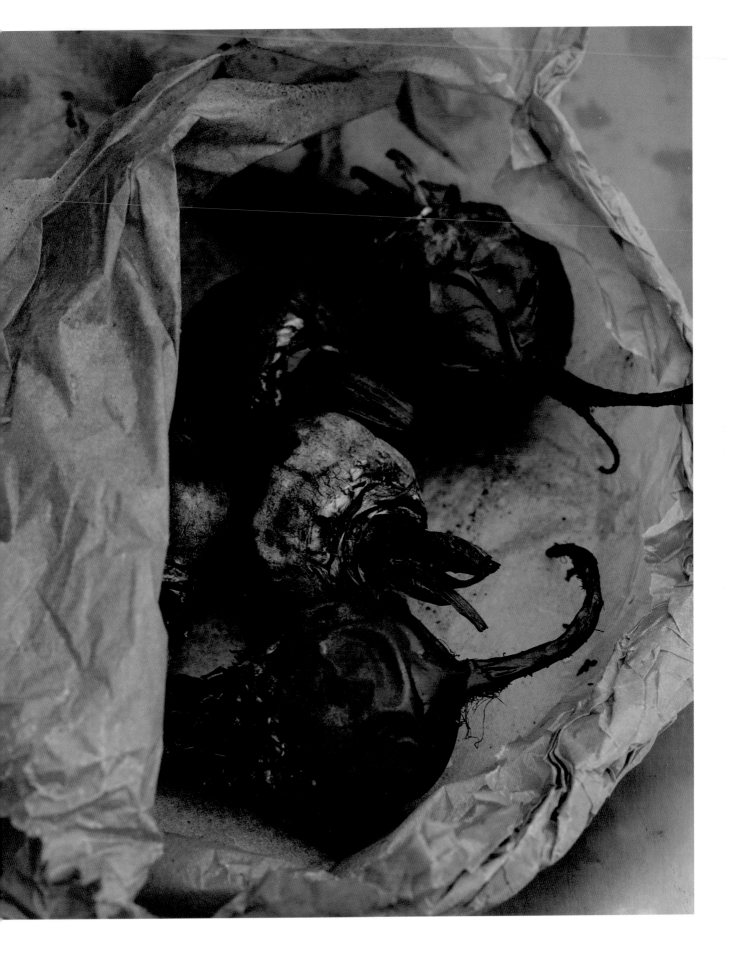

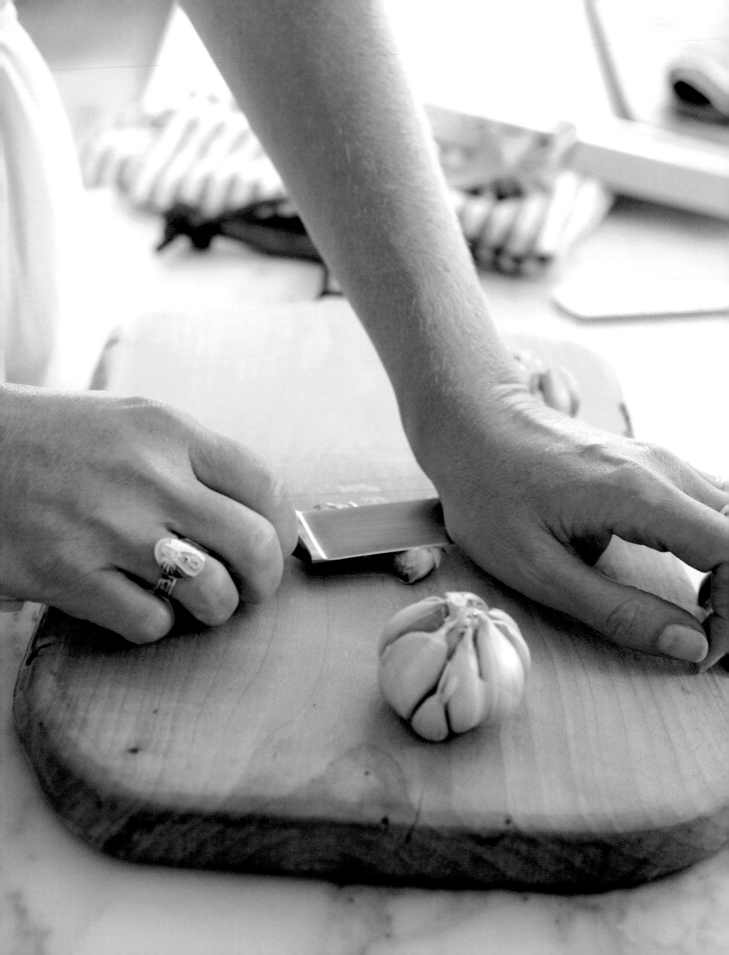

Mexican Black Beans

QUICK / VEGAN

Serves 2 or 3

The fifteen minutes required to simmer black beans with a few simple aromatics gives them incredible flavor and is totally worth the effort. My kids love to eat these with rice and guac (don't forget the hot sauce!), and I love them on the Tex-Mex Bowl (page 77).

1 (14-ounce) can organic black beans, undrained

4 cilantro sprigs

1 garlic clove, crushed

A pinch of kosher salt

Combine all the ingredients in a small saucepan and simmer over low heat for 15 to 20 minutes. Be sure to simmer the beans long enough that they're not watery.

Serve warm or at room temperature, or store in an airtight container in the fridge for later use, up to 5 days.

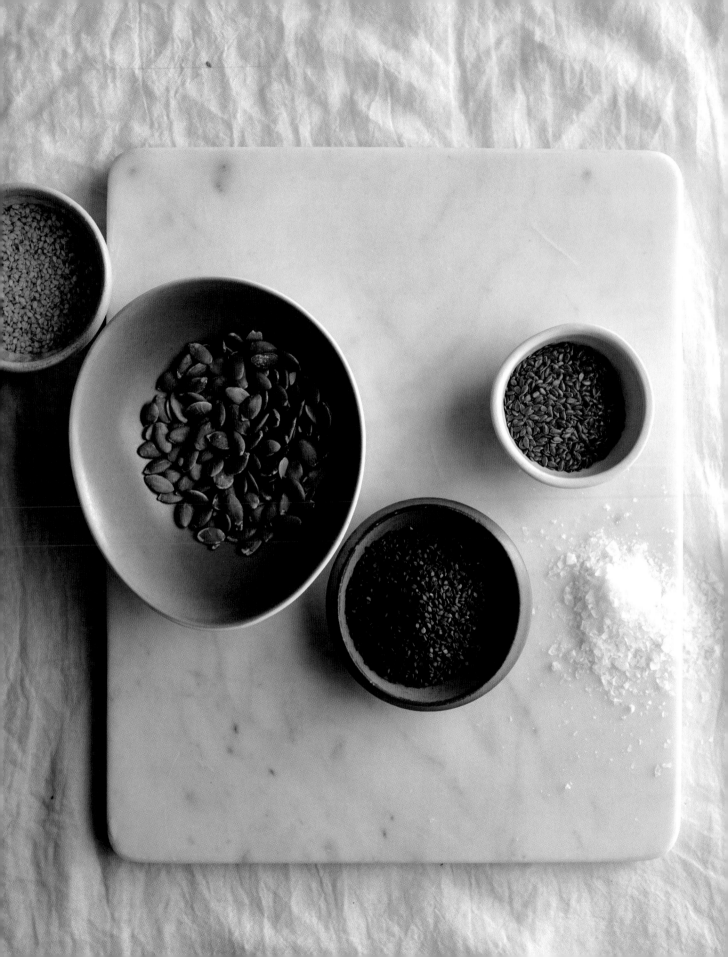

Seed Cracker

VEGAN

Makes 1 roughly 8×11-inch cracker

Chef Magnus Nilsson made a version of this 100 percent grain- and gluten-free cracker when he came to visit the goop test kitchen, and it blew my mind. I use it as a base for cleaned-up avocado toasts (page 16) or dip pieces into hummus for an easy afternoon snack.

½ cup flaxseeds

1 tablespoon arrowroot powder

¼ teaspoon kosher salt

3 tablespoons black sesame seeds

3 tablespoons white sesame seeds

3 tablespoons hulled pepitas

1 cup boiling water

Flaky sea salt

Preheat the oven to 320°F.

In a medium bowl, mix together all the ingredients except the flaky salt. Let sit for 15 minutes to firm up.

Lay a large sheet of parchment paper on your work surface and use a spatula to scrape the seed mixture onto the paper. Top with another piece of parchment and use a rolling pin to roll the mixture into an 8×11, ¼-inch-thick sheet.

Transfer to a baking sheet and carefully peel off the top layer of parchment (go slowly, as a few seeds may stick to it). Sprinkle with flaky salt and bake for 45 minutes.

Let cool, then break the cracker into large pieces and store in an airtight container for up to 1 week.

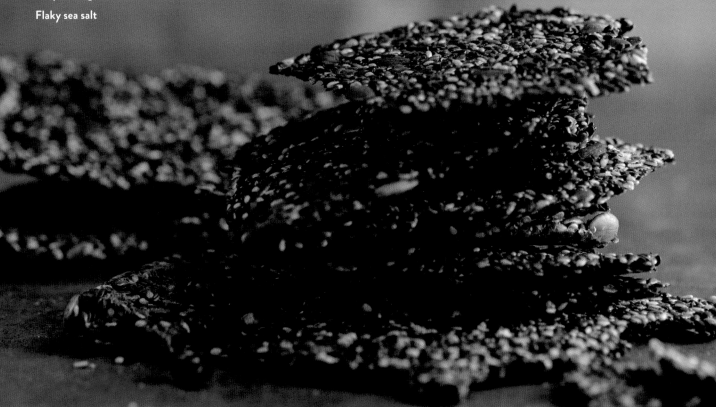

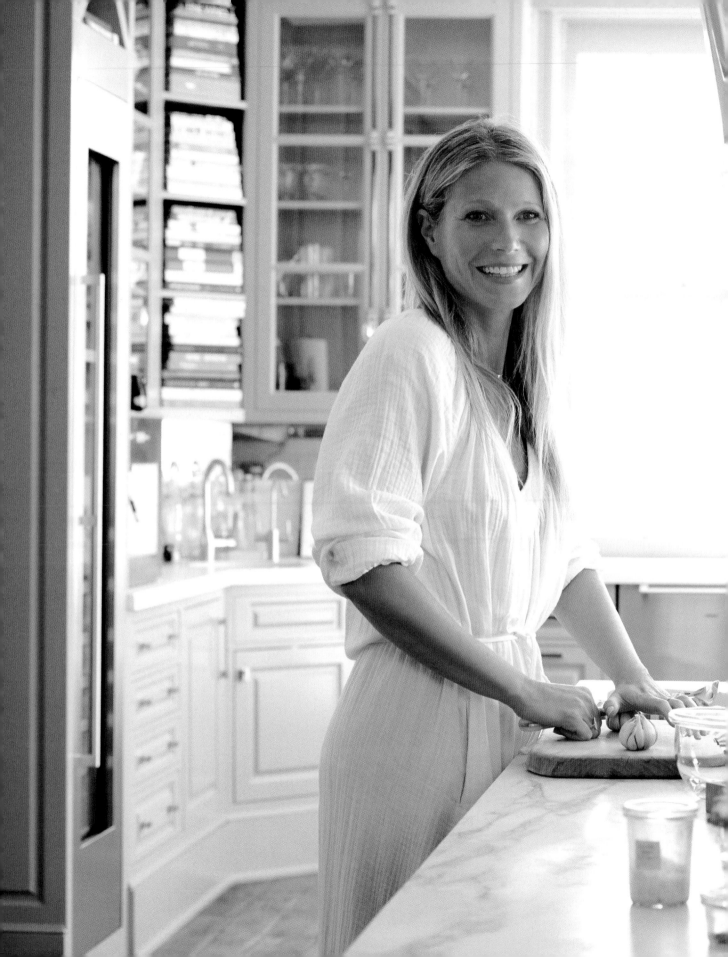

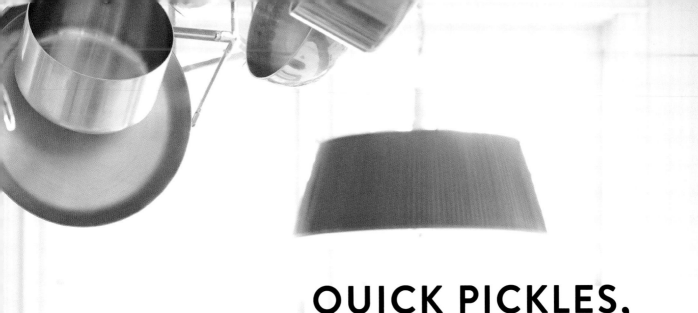

QUICK PICKLES, 3 WAYS

Pickles are such a great way to add flavor and texture to a dish. All three of these pickles use a similar brine, but I changed up the aromatics a little in each one. Feel free to play around with what you use to flavor the brine—spices like cinnamon sticks, fennel seeds, or turmeric would all taste good.

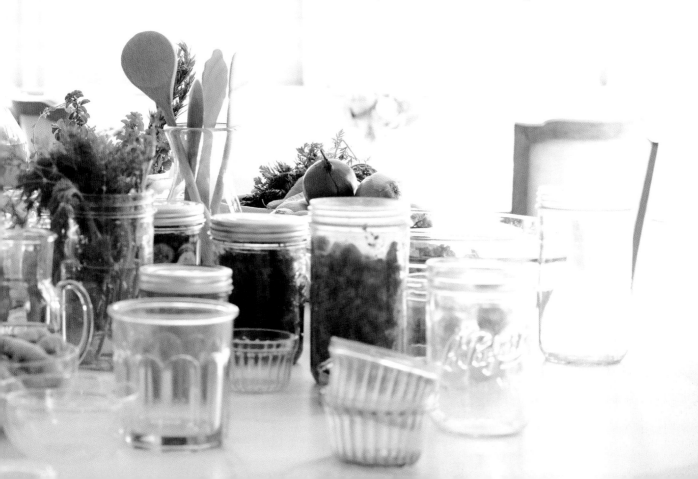

Pickled Red Onions

QUICK / VEGAN

Makes about 2 cups

Even people who say they don't like onions will like these pickled onions.

1 medium red onion, thinly sliced

¾ cup water

1 tablespoon whole black peppercorns

1 teaspoon kosher salt

1 garlic clove, crushed

1 star anise pod

½ teaspoon coriander seeds

1¼ cups apple cider vinegar

4 drops of liquid stevia (not a stevia-based sweetener)

Put the onion in a medium bowl and set aside.

Combine the water, peppercorns, salt, garlic, star anise, and coriander in a small saucepan and bring to a boil. Remove from the heat, add the vinegar and stevia, then pour directly over the onions.

Let cool, then refrigerate. The pickles are ready to eat as soon as they're cool. These should last for a few days stored in a covered jar or bowl in the refrigerator.

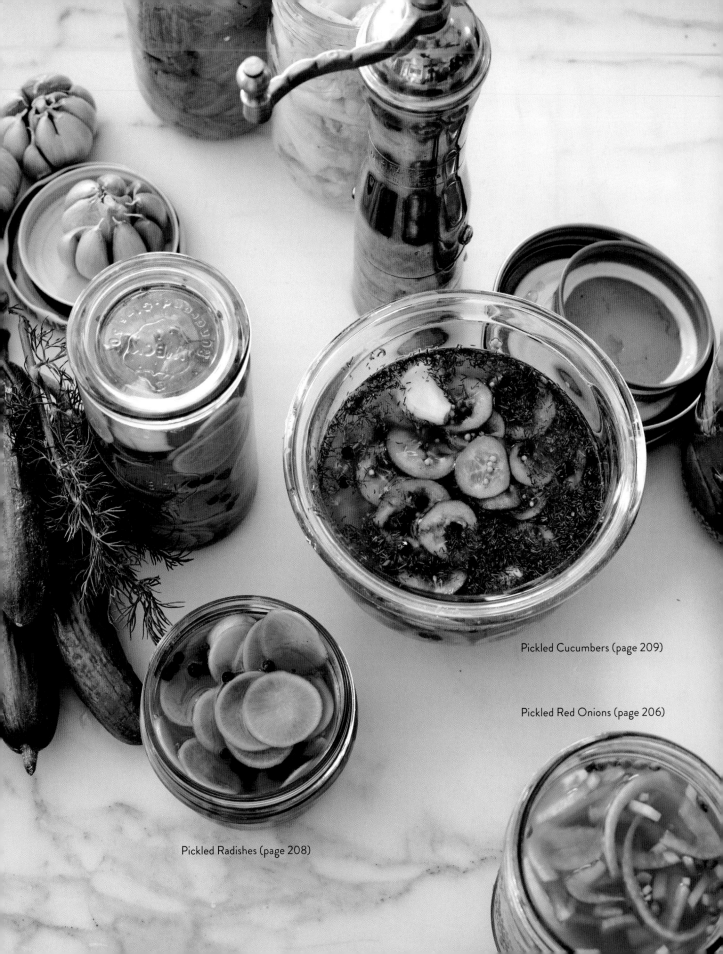

Pickled Cucumbers (page 209)

Pickled Red Onions (page 206)

Pickled Radishes (page 208)

Pickled Radishes

QUICK / VEGAN

Makes about 2 cups

Mexican oregano is the key to making these taste like authentic taqueria-style pickles. (This recipe would work great with carrots, too.)

1 bunch of radishes, thinly sliced

¾ cup water

1 tablespoon whole black peppercorns

1 teaspoon kosher salt

3 garlic cloves, smashed

½ teaspoon dried Mexican oregano

1 bay leaf

¼ teaspoon chili flakes (optional)

1¼ cups apple cider vinegar

4 drops of liquid stevia (not a stevia-based sweetener)

Put the radishes in a medium bowl and set aside.

Combine the water, peppercorns, salt, garlic, oregano, bay leaf, and chili flakes (if using) in a small saucepan and bring to a boil. Remove from the heat, add the vinegar and stevia, then pour directly over the radishes.

Let cool, then refrigerate. The pickles are ready to eat as soon as they're cool. These should last for a few days stored in a covered jar or bowl in the refrigerator.

Pickled Cucumbers

QUICK / VEGAN

Makes about 2 cups

These are nice on top of a burger, but I love them as little snackers on their own.

4 Persian cucumbers, sliced about ¼ inch thick

¾ cup water

1 tablespoon whole black peppercorns

1 teaspoon kosher salt

3 garlic cloves, smashed

1 teaspoon mustard seeds

1 tablespoon chopped fresh dill

4 drops of liquid stevia (not a stevia-based sweetener)

1¼ cups apple cider vinegar

Put the cucumbers in a medium bowl and set aside.

Combine the water, peppercorns, salt, garlic, and mustard seeds in a small saucepan and bring to a boil. Remove from the heat, add the dill, stevia, and vinegar, then pour directly over the cucumbers.

Let cool, then refrigerate. The pickles are ready to eat as soon as they're cool. These should last for a few days stored in a covered jar or bowl in the refrigerator.

Chia Seed Jam

VEGAN

Makes about 1 cup

There always seems to be a surplus of blueberries in my fridge. This blueberry jam solves the problem of using them before they turn. (I know, good problem to have.) The trick is to let the blueberries reduce a bit so the jam sweetens up without added sugars or sweeteners.

1 cup blueberries

2 tablespoons fresh lemon juice

3 tablespoons chia seeds

In a small saucepan, combine blueberries and lemon juice. Cook over medium-high heat, stirring frequently, for 5 to 6 minutes, until the blueberries start to break down and have released most of their liquid.

Using an immersion blender, blend the blueberries directly in the pot until smooth. Simmer over medium-high heat for 4 to 5 minutes, until the blueberry puree thickens a little bit.

Transfer the blueberry puree to a small bowl or small jar. Stir in the chia seeds and let sit for 10 minutes before using, or let cool completely, cover, and store in the fridge for up to 5 days.

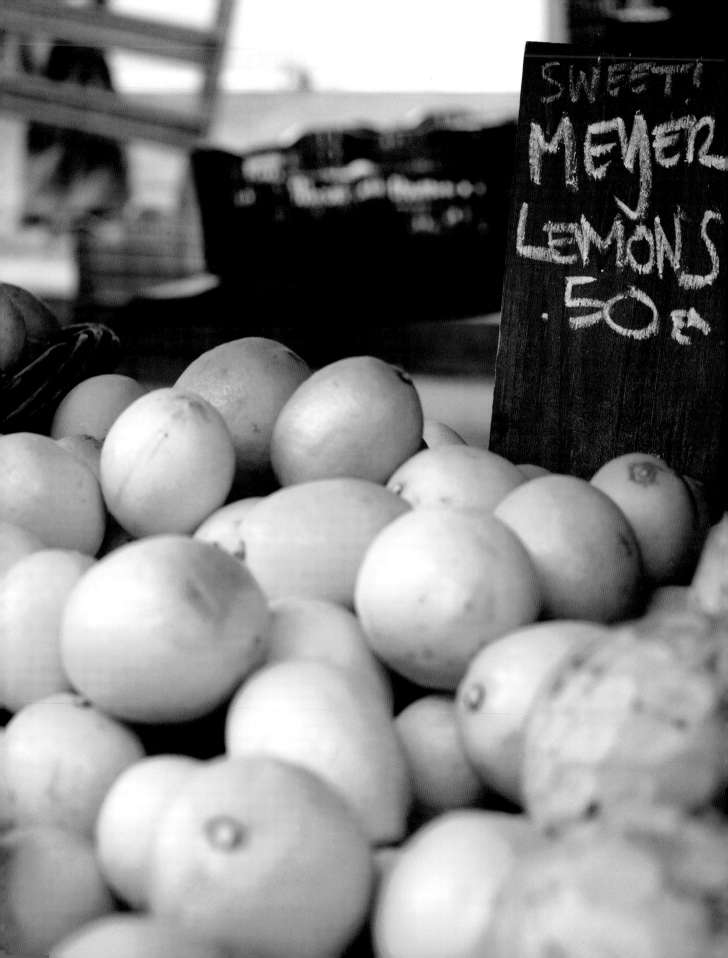

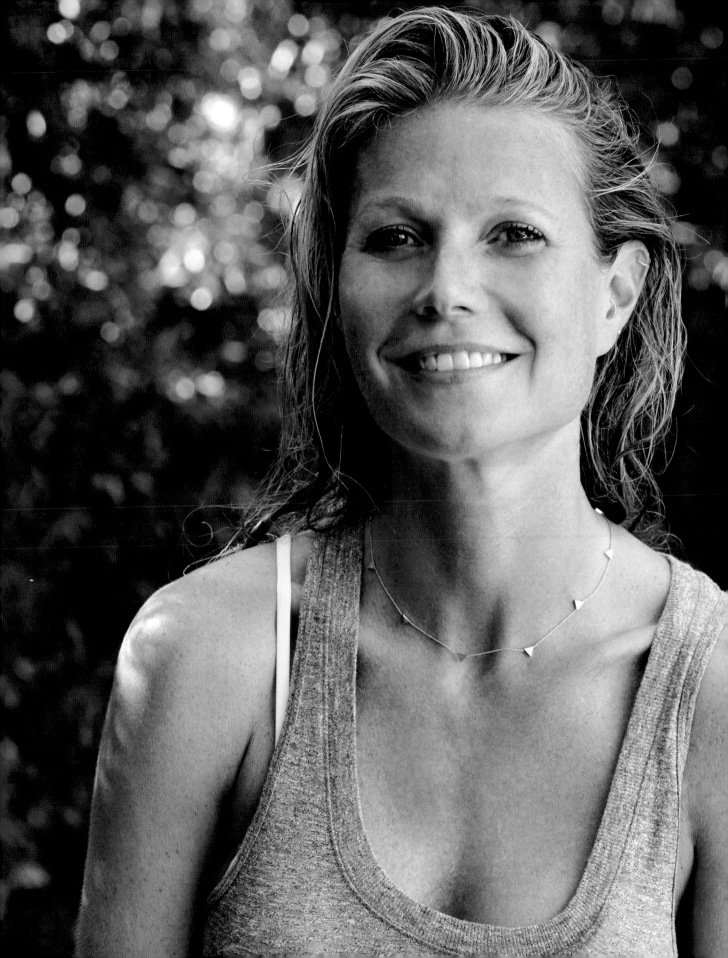

PART II

HEALING CLEANSES

Nearly all my doctors over the years have had a food-first philosophy in common. Here I'm sharing interviews with six practitioners who inspire me, each on their respective area of expertise, and all with an eye toward eating to maximize our health.

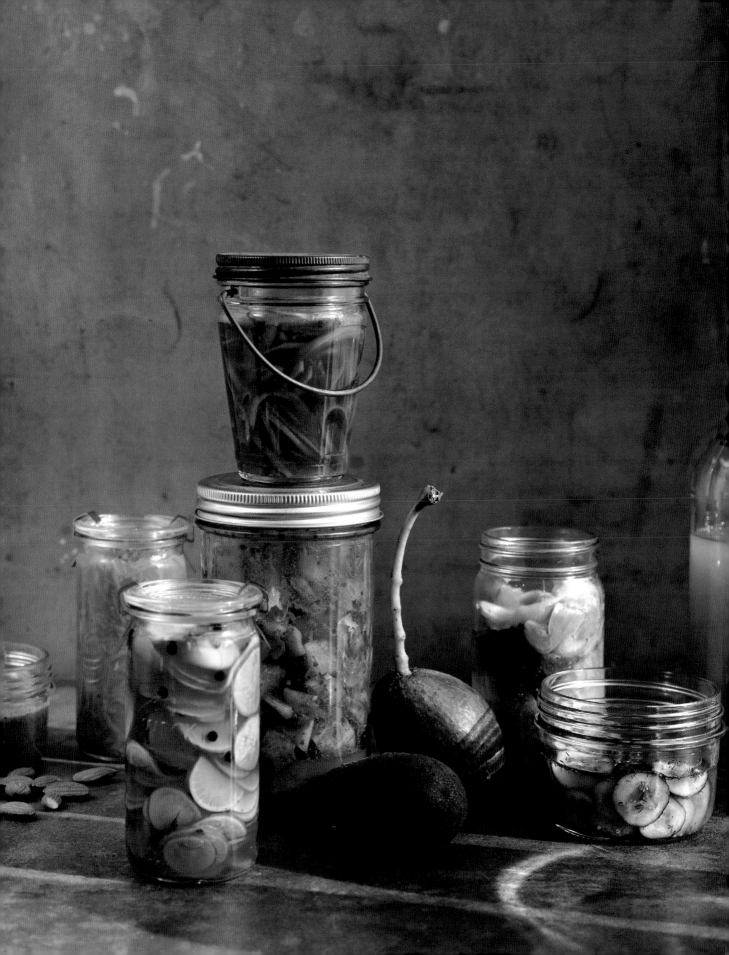

FAT FLUSH

Here's what I know from talking to friends who have felt betrayed by their bodies after having kids or hitting a certain age, and from sitting down with some of the most cutting-edge hormone and nutrition experts: The equations around the health of our metabolism, the balance of our hormones, how we gain or lose weight, how we process fat and where we store it, and ultimately our relationship to food and our bodies is infinitely complex and about much more than digits on a scale or how we look. For help decoding it all, enter Dr. Taz Bhatia, an Atlanta-based, board-certified integrative medicine physician, and author of *Super Woman Rx*, who takes an East-meets-West, holistic approach to matters of metabolism.

A Q&A WITH TAZ BHATIA, MD

Q: What's typically behind weight loss resistance?

A: Weight loss is tricky, especially for women. Doctors and researchers today are realizing that weight loss and weight gain have to be treated comprehensively and holistically to really gain tangible results. Weight loss resistance occurs when the classic balance of "calories in, calories out" no longer works. Many patients will say they went back to restricting their calories to lose that stubborn 5 or 10 pounds, and it did not work like it once had. There are a number of reasons this may be the case:

First, hormone balance in women plays a role in our metabolic weight or ability to gain or lose weight. Thyroid, insulin, estrogen, progesterone, testosterone, and cortisol are all hormones that can affect someone's ability to lose weight.

Gut function is another factor that impacts weight gain. Declining pancreatic function, resulting in a loss of digestive enzymes, and declining levels of stomach acid and shifts in the microbiome are all potential causes of weight gain. Additionally, food intolerances can contribute to this equation, making weight loss all the more challenging.

Nutritional deficiencies are a factor, as they affect weight, among many other aspects of health. I see a lot of vitamin B deficiencies in women who struggle with weight loss resistance. Low levels of vitamin D, iron, magnesium, and fatty acids can also come into play. Fatty acid deficiencies affect how we metabolize fat—instead of using fat effectively, we may hold on to it or not break it down to where the body can use it. This can cause blood sugar levels to fluctuate, which gives way to food cravings and can contribute to insulin resistance patterns (more on this in a moment).

Q: Which hormones are most likely to get thrown out of whack, and why?

A: The hormones most likely to be thrown off include cortisol (the stress hormone produced by the adrenal glands) and insulin (a hormone made in the pancreas in response to food). There are a number of reasons for this: Many of us live highly stressful lives, and that drives our bodies to produce more cortisol, for longer periods of time; after a point, this affects blood sugar and insulin regulation. Insulin irregularity can trigger fat storage, which can lead to stubborn belly weight, back fat, and general weight gain.

Insulin is meant to help the body absorb glucose and use it for energy. Insulin resistance occurs when cells don't respond properly to insulin, which prompts the body to produce more insulin, while blood sugar levels continue to rise. Unfortunately, once that switch is flipped and the body becomes insulin resistant, it's tougher to reverse it. Studies often show that to really affect weight loss, a total reset of insulin is required, which can take 3 to 6 weeks.

Leptin and ghrelin—known as the hunger hormones—also play a role. In short, leptin decreases appetite and ghrelin signals hunger. An imbalance of these two hormones can throw off insulin and cortisol. One issue I see with women who consistently don't get enough sleep is that they have high levels of ghrelin, and they don't produce leptin in the right amount, which can make you hunger resistant—in other words, you don't recognize when you're full anymore. Stress, coupled with lack of sleep, can cause cortisol to spike as well.

Thyroid hormone is critical. When the thyroid is sluggish, the body typically stores more estrogen rather than using it and then getting rid of it, which can cause weight gain. (High estrogen, called estrogen dominance, can trigger or worsen insulin resistance.) An overactive thyroid can actually be associated with weight gain, too, because this dysfunction can throw metabolism off. Nutritional deficiencies can negatively impact thyroid health—particularly low levels of iron, iodine, selenium, and zinc. And if the issue is not super severe, patients can often reset the thyroid through diet.

For the thyroid to function effectively, you need your adrenal glands to be functioning effectively. This goes back to stress and cortisol—so many of us are burning the candle at both ends, which means the adrenals have to work harder, the thyroid has to work harder, and our hormone balance often suffers. It's all interconnected.

Q: Is there testing that you typically recommend for people coming to you for weight loss resistance?

A: We conduct a full battery of testing at my practice, CentreSpring MD, including testing all hormone and nutrient levels, for food allergies and food intolerances, and stool tests to assess microbiome function.

When it comes to hormone testing, you might have heard that your hormone levels vary depending on where you are in your menstrual cycle. This is true, but there are boundaries regardless—for instance, I don't like to see estrogen over 200 (this is estrogen dominance) or progesterone below 0.5. Here are some hormone highlights and ideal value ranges to be aware of:

- Thyroid-stimulating hormone (TSH): 1–2 mIU/L
- Free triiodothyronine (free T3): 3–5 pg/ml
- Estradiol (a form of estrogen): 50–150 pg/ml
- Estrone (a form of estrogen): less than 150 pg/ml
- Progesterone: 0.5–2 ng/ml
- C-peptide (a marker of pre–insulin resistance): 1–3 ng/ml
- Leptin: 5–15 ng/ml

You can also get your fasting insulin level checked, which can tell you if your insulin is too high (over 5 ng/l or MG/DL when fasting). You can get your cortisol checked with a spit test—for the most accurate picture, you'll do this throughout the day (a healthy range is 10 to 20 ug/dl in the morning, and drops to 3 to 4 ug/dl in the afternoon).

It's easier to have a stool test ordered than hormone testing—stool tests are typically covered by lab insurance and can be done by conventional doctors, so you don't need to see a functional MD, necessarily. With stool tests, one thing I look for is fecal fats—when the body is spilling fat globules it's a sign that you aren't digesting fat well, which, as mentioned, can affect blood sugar levels.

Depending on the patient, more complex gut tests might be ordered to check for microbiome dysfunctions—e.g., Candida, small intestinal bacterial overgrowth (SIBO), enzyme deficiency, or other outliers like parasites.

In terms of nutrient levels, some key ranges I look for are:

- Vitamin D: 50–70 ng/ml
- B$_{12}$: over 500 pg/ml
- Ferritin (iron): 50–70 ng/ml
- Magnesium: greater than 2.2 mg/ml

Q: Can a cleanse actually help kick-start your metabolism and help you shed pounds? Are there any detox add-ons you recommend?

A: Yes—the essential purpose of a detox is to give the liver and the gut a resting period, reset blood sugar and insulin irregularity, and give the body a nutrient superboost to help improve metabolism.

If you don't get your diet right, no detox add-ons are going to make a difference. But to complement a good diet, I like steaming, infrared saunas, whirlpools, and Epsom salt soaks.

Q: What does your protocol for weight loss look like?

A: My protocol for weight loss focuses on three main steps, each lasting a week.

- The first week is focused on detoxification and hormone balancing. This includes removing grain, dairy, sugar, and red meat.

- The second week is about balancing and improving digestion. During this week, we add gut-balancing foods like probiotic-rich kefir or kombucha, bone broth, and digestive enzymes and probiotics.

- The third week is more focused on movement, exercise, and sleep. Learning to increase heart rate, build muscle, and stretch can all be components of weight loss.

Q: Can you go into more detail on foods to steer clear of?

A: High-sugar foods, sodas, sweet drinks are obvious no's.

Refined sugar, added sugars, processed sugars—monk fruit, stevia, sugar, honey, agave—all of that should be under 25 grams a day, or below 3 teaspoons. Lower is ideal.

Excessive consumption of fruit can be an issue as well. The sugar in fruit, although natural, can be just another addition to an already ricocheting blood sugar level. I suggest sticking to one serving of fruit per day, and picking lower-sugar fruit, like berries (as opposed to bananas and citrus). Apples are also a good choice, as the fiber they contain brings the glycemic index down. If you have Candida overgrowth (which many of my patients with insulin resistance and weight loss resistance do), you should skip fruit, as the sugar feeds the yeast.

If you're counting carbs, you likely want to be under 150 total carbs per day. But if you're an athlete or otherwise super active, you may need more. If you have a mood disorder or severe anxiety, be aware that dropping your carbs too low can worsen these symptoms.

Q: What about good ingredients to add?

A: Adding in MCT (medium-chain triglycerides) oils in the form of coconut oil and other healthy fats like avocado, olive oil, and ghee can help to better balance insulin and keep blood sugar levels stable. Getting enough fat helps you to feel satiated and cut sugar cravings down.

Superfoods like greens, seeds, and nut butters help to boost antioxidants. Fiber and protein are key for energy.

Bitter foods like artichokes, radishes, and dandelion root help the digestive process by activating the production of hydrochloric acid and digestive enzymes. You can also take squeeze bitters before eating.

Apple cider vinegar is easy to add to foods (like salad dressings), and some patients report that it helps with weight management, particularly belly fat.

The first few days of a cleanse, if you're going through sugar withdrawal, you might feel the urge to eat even if you're not really hungry. Sipping on green tea or decaf tea can help blunt the craving. You can also try drinking mini tonics made with ingredients like dandelion, celery, or turmeric throughout the day.

It's less "natural," but people report that chewing gum or sucking on a mint prevents them from feeling like they need to snack constantly.

Q: Which supplements do you recommend?

A: For weight loss, I recommend a multi-B vitamin, as it is essential for women's health. B vitamins are involved in estrogen metabolism, as well as progesterone, thyroid, and adrenal health. They play a role with almost every hormone, and deficiencies can correlate with estrogen buildup and cortisol spikes.

Probiotics can be beneficial for overall microbiome health and are ideally tailored to your personal health. For many of my patients with weight resistance and correlated Candida issues, I recommend probiotics higher in *Lactobacillus* and *Bifidobacterium* strains.

Digestive enzymes with ox bile and lipase can help the body metabolize fat.

Q: What about exercise and other lifestyle changes?

A: Once insulin resistance sets in, daily movement is usually needed for approximately 45 minutes per day. For at least 20 of those minutes, you want your heart rate at double your resting rate.

Adding weight training, at least 2 days per week, is also great because the body's metabolic response helps with blood sugar balance and burning energy more efficiently.

But if stress levels are high—then yoga, Pilates, and sometimes swimming are often better options. For patients who are in danger of being further fatigued, injured, or quitting, I like to focus on food, resetting the gut, getting adequate sleep, and bringing cortisol down. Once cortisol is in check, then it might be time to consider higher-powered exercise.

Overall, sleep is crucial, especially for women because of our cycling. Not getting sufficient sleep can affect hormone signaling (cortisol in particular), causing weight gain, among other health issues.

Q: Once the body is reset, what's important to keeping everything in balance and maintaining a healthy weight?

A: Doing more of the same: Maintaining good sleep, food, and exercise habits while keeping your gut balanced are key to maintaining your weight.

A daily fasting interval of 14 hours, and a weekly fast, can be helpful as well, and continues the benefits of a softer, less involved detox. Keeping close to a 14-hour window (including overnight) in which you're not eating helps to support digestion. Between meals, try to avoid grazing constantly, and give your body at least 4 hours to digest and break everything down.

A weekly fast doesn't have to mean only drinking water for a day. Some people will go meatless, all-veggie, and sugar-free for one day a week as a way of cutting back what might build up in the system.

You also want to be sure you're sweating regularly and having good bowel movements (going to the bathroom at least once a day).

Q: Do you see an emotional component to metabolism and weight?

A: In Chinese medicine, there is thought to be an emotional root to all energy meridian imbalances. People in pain, stress, or trauma, or who have lost their spark or passion, will sometimes eat and use food as a way to medicate. They are so disconnected that they usually don't realize they're doing this. A lot of us can relate to this—raiding the pantry when we're just bored or stressed but not really hungry.

We have to learn to recognize our emotional cues and how we're actually feeling. If we don't understand our emotional and mental landscape, we can have the best plan in the world but still sabotage it. All the chemistry and talk of hormones and gut balance is a moot point if our relationship to food and our bodies is dysfunctional.

Changing your emotional landscape is the hardest and probably the most important work. There is no quick fix. But what might help? Try checking in with your body, spending time in nature, developing a spiritual connection, taking time to care for yourself, doing work you love.

The Food Shortlist

BEST TO AVOID

- Dairy (ghee is okay)
- Gluten
- Limit red meat
- Refined sugar (limit fruit sugars)

GOOD TO ADD

- Apple cider vinegar
- Avocado
- Coconut oil
- Fermented foods
- Greens
- Nut butters
- Olive oil
- Seeds

The goopified Menu

	MONDAY	TUESDAY	WEDNESDAY	THURSDAY	FRIDAY	SATURDAY	SUNDAY
BREAKFAST	Veggie Scramble (page 19)	Seed Cracker with Egg & Avocado (page 16)	Sweet Buckwheat Porridge (page 25)	Quinoa Cereal with Freeze-Dried Berries (page 24)	Kale Kuku Soccata (page 8)	Breakfast Dal (page 11)	Seed Cracker with Smoked Salmon & Avocado (page 15)
LUNCH	Nori Salad Roll (page 93)	Teriyaki Bowl (page 73)	Miso Soup (page 47)	Kimchi Chicken Lettuce Cups (page 83)	Crunchy Summer Rolls (page 91)	Garden Salad with Aquafaba Ranch Dressing (page 59)	Coconut Chicken Soup (page 41)
DINNER	Sheet Pan Chicken Curry (page 119)	Peruvian Chicken Cauli Rice Soup (page 44)	Fish Tacos on Jicama "Tortillas" (page 99)	Black Rice with Braised Chicken Thighs (page 109)	White Bean & Zucchini Burgers (page 124)	Chicken & Cabbage Dim Sum (page 145)	Mediterranean Salmon en Papillote (page 113)

A FEW GO-TO SNACKS:

- Seed Cracker (page 203) with almond butter
- Seed Cracker with avocado and sauerkraut
- Half an avocado with sea salt and lime juice

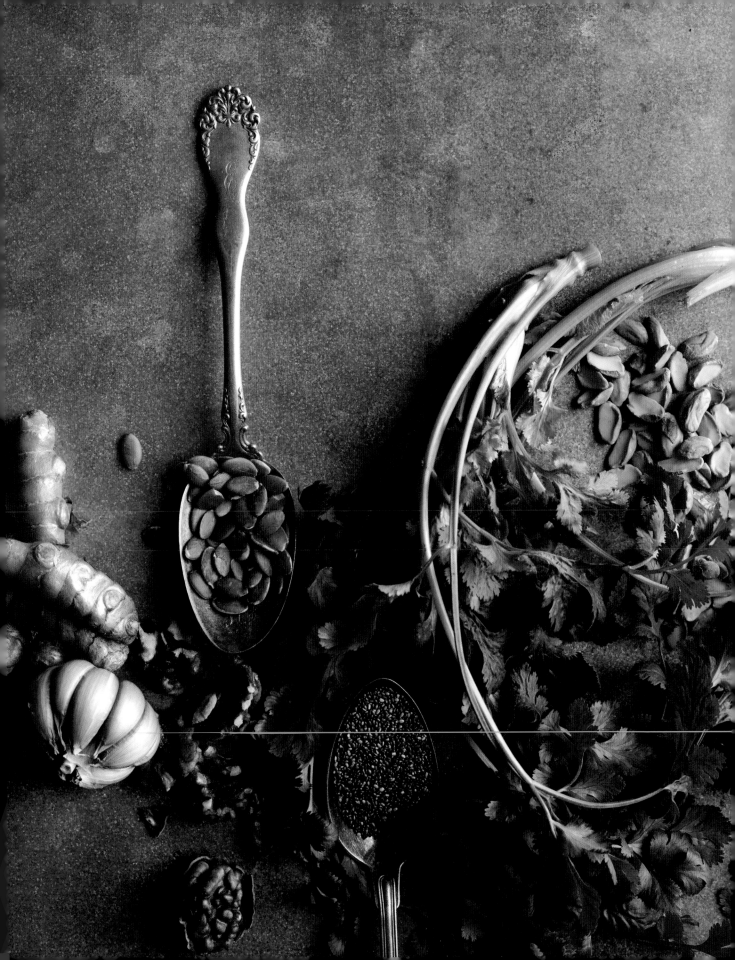

HEAVY METAL DETOX

Southern California–based Dr. James Novak sees a number of patients concerned with heavy metal toxicity (among other hard-to-solve symptoms). There's still a lot that science doesn't know about heavy metals. Novak explains that we're all exposed to these toxins on a daily basis, but very few people require aggressive treatment because of it. With that in mind, he shares tips for decreasing your toxic load in the first place and for supporting the body's natural mechanisms for getting rid of heavy metals.

A Q&A WITH JAMES NOVAK, MD

Q: What are the major sources of heavy metal exposure?

A: It is impossible to live in the modern world without exposure to a multitude of toxins. Toxins are ubiquitous in the air we breathe, the water we drink, and the food we eat. Fortunately for us, the mind/body is a self-regulating, self-healing system that is well-equipped with multiple homeostatic systems to deal with this problem constantly (assuming it is not completely overloaded).

Heavy metal exposure, more specifically, is ubiquitous in our everyday environment. People are exposed regularly to nano-sized aluminum from geoengineering aerosols, as well as from cooking pots and antiperspirants. The primary exposure sources of inorganic mercury are mercury amalgams in teeth, organic mercury in fish high in the food chain (shark, tuna, swordfish), and high-fructose corn syrup (which may be contaminated with mercury and is a staple in processed foods). People can be exposed to arsenic in rice and chicken. The amount of arsenic ingested from rice may be minimized by cooking with lots of water (a ratio of about 6 to 10 parts water to 1 part rice). The amount of arsenic ingested with chicken can be minimized by consuming organic chicken. Shellfish can contain cadmium, as well as other toxic compounds, depending on the watershed from which it is harvested. Lead can get stored in our bones from previous exposure to fumes from leaded gasoline.

Q: Why do you consider heavy metals a health concern?

A: Heavy metals can denature enzymes, disrupt normal cellular metabolism, and cause oxidative stress. For example, mercury molecules in the mitochondria can cause free radical reactions, which may put stress on cellular antioxidant defenses and weaken resistance to other cellular stressors such as bacteria, viruses, and other toxins.

Q: When do heavy metals become an issue? What are the related symptoms, and can you test for toxicity?

A: Research suggests that newborn babies actually inherit a toxic load from their mothers, so heavy metal toxicity is a health concern that everyone should be aware of. But until people get to a point where their compensation mechanisms—their cellular detoxification enzymes—are saturated, they usually do not experience overt symptoms.

Because many heavy metals are chronic neurologic, endocrine, and immune disruptors that can undermine the mechanisms by which these systems self-regulate and heal, there is a wide range of potential symptoms. Symptoms of advanced heavy metal toxicity can include fatigue, cognitive impairment, palpitations, muscle weakness, and dizziness, depending on which tissue compartment the heavy metals have accumulated in in the body.

Probably the best test for heavy metal toxicity is provided by Quicksilver Scientific. It reveals normal mineral metabolism along with the standard toxic elements, e.g., levels of lead, cadmium, mercury, arsenic, etc. Additionally, the test speciates the mercury into organic and inorganic components, which is helpful because knowing the relative amount of each form gives you a better idea of the degree of toxicity (more organic mercury is worse because it absorbs into body tissues more readily). Since it simultaneously tests hair, urine, and blood samples, it can also help show whether detox systems in the body are working to eliminate toxins properly, or whether accumulation is progressing due to faulty elimination.

Q: What does your typical heavy metal detox protocol look like?

A: I think everyone needs to approach supporting the body's heavy metal detoxification as an ongoing lifestyle. A minority of severely affected people may need aggressive treatment with intravenous chelation under the supervision of a doctor. The word "chelation" is derived from the Greek word "Chele," meaning "claw." Intravenous administration of a chelator such as EDTA or DMPS two to three times a week grabs heavy metals electromagnetically between the molecular "claws" of the chelator, and transports them to the liver and kidneys for elimination. But the vast majority of people can benefit greatly from a simpler lifestyle approach.

For more support, a gentle detox protocol over a 3- to 6-month period can be helpful:

STEP ONE:
REMOVE THE SOURCE

Remove or minimize ongoing sources of exposure. This means avoiding processed foods, and fruits and vegetables with pesticide and herbicide contamination; fresh, organic fruits, vegetables, and herbs are best. High-mercury fish (like shark, tuna, swordfish), as well as shellfish, should be avoided. Meat and fowl should be organic, preferably pasture-fed. If you're eating rice, I recommend basmati, jasmine, and Himalayan.

Unfiltered tap water should be avoided. The best sources of water—free of fluoride, heavy metals, and organic pollutants—are obtained from spring water (I like Mountain Valley Spring Water, which comes in glass bottles) or home reverse osmosis filters, distillers, or atmospheric water generators.

Aluminum cooking vessels should be avoided—stainless steel is okay—as well as antiperspirants containing aluminum. Glass containers should be used for drinking water.

Some people may remove mercury amalgams gradually. Use a biological dentist trained in safe mercury removal.

STEP TWO:
SUPPORT DETOXIFICATION

In general, we can support the body's detox mechanisms in the skin, kidneys, and gastrointestinal tract: Sweating, either by exercise or far infrared sauna, can help remove toxins through the skin. Adequate hydration can enhance renal clearance of toxins. And proper nutrition can support the removal of toxins from the tissues, the processing of toxins in the liver, and the binding of toxins in the intestinal tract for ultimate excretion in the stool.

More specifically, heavy metals such as lead, mercury, and arsenic are excreted from the cells by special protein structures called metallothionein enzymes. These structures require minerals such as zinc, copper, selenium, and magnesium to function properly. Eating foods rich in these minerals can aid these enzyme systems in releasing tissue toxins into the blood. Good sources include nuts and seeds, legumes, Atlantic seaweeds, leafy green vegetables, fulvic and humic mineral supplements, sea salt, and herbs such as burdock root, horsetail, and red clover. Regular consumption of cilantro can also aid in the mobilization of heavy metals from tissue compartments.

Once in the blood, the toxic substances are carried to the gastrointestinal tract, where they undergo a two-phase process for transformation and eventual elimination from the body. The initial process, phase one, involves oxidation and hydrolysis of the toxic substance via the p450 enzymes in the liver. This process converts the toxic substance into a form that will eventually be easier to excrete. Cruciferous vegetables—such as broccoli, cabbage, cauliflower, and Brussels sprouts—can support this process.

The second phase of detoxification involves a process called conjugation, where another compound is attached to the toxin to make it easier to excrete. A variety of biochemical mechanisms can be involved at this point—sulfation, glucuronidation, acetylation, methylation, glutathione conjugation. Sulfur-rich foods such as eggs, garlic, onions, leeks, shallots, and cruciferous vegetables may all help facilitate this process.

When the conjugated toxins are ready for excretion, they flow with the bile into the intestines. Cholagogues, such as curcumin, can help stimulate the flow of bile into the intestines.

Once the toxins enter the intestinal tract, we don't want them to be reabsorbed into the bloodstream. Eating bulking foods such as citrus pectin, seaweed alginates, and mucilaginous foods (like flax and chia seeds) may help prevent reabsorption of metals that have already been eliminated as they pass down the intestinal tract.

In terms of supplements, some people may take iodine supplements to support heavy metal excretion.

Q: What do you recommend for patients if this doesn't work?

A: Depending on the patient, I may incorporate additional elements into the protocol, like a multimineral, cilantro tincture, or fulvic acid (to promote tissue release); n-acetyl cysteine (to promote liver conjugation/excretion); and PectaClear (modified citrus pectin/seaweed alginate) with chlorella (as intestinal binders).

For those individuals who need a more aggressive approach, I may prescribe a cycle of oral chelation using DMSA (dimercaptosuccinic acid) capsules, 3 days on, 11 days off, until retesting demonstrates the desired improvement. I usually will retest for heavy metals after 3 to 4 months of treatment.

A potent oral chelator, Irminix (emeramide) by EmeraMed, is undergoing regulatory approval in Europe and will likely be available as a doctor prescription in the next year or two; it will also likely become the gold standard of care. This chelator is absorbed orally and crosses the blood-brain barrier. A 2-week course of 300mg per day has been shown to eliminate mercury residues from the body. Once mercury residues are reduced, Irminix can then start to eliminate arsenic, lead, and other toxic metals based on the degree of electromagnetic attraction it has for each element.

The Food Shortlist

BEST TO AVOID

- Added sugars
- Grains with mycotoxin residue
- High-mercury fish/shellfish
- Non-organic fruits and vegetables
- Non-organic meat/chicken
- Processed foods
- Toxic oils
- Unfiltered tap water

GOOD TO ADD

- Adequate spring/reverse osmosis/distilled water
- Alliums (garlic, onions, leeks, shallots)
- Bitter greens (dandelion, beet greens, chicory, turmeric)
- Cilantro
- Cruciferous vegetables
- Eggs
- Leafy green vegetables
- Nuts and seeds
- Seaweeds
- Sea salts

The goopified Menu

	MONDAY	TUESDAY	WEDNESDAY	THURSDAY	FRIDAY	SATURDAY	SUNDAY
BREAKFAST	Chlorella Smoothie (page 166)	Cauliflower, Pea & Turmeric Soccata (page 7)	Kale Kuku Soccata (page 8)	Poached Eggs over Sautéed Greens (page 22)	Easy Frittata (page 21)	Strawberry Cauliflower Smoothie (page 163)	Breakfast Dal (page 11)
LUNCH	Curry Chicken Lettuce Cups (page 84)	Clean Carrot Soup (page 33)	Miso Soup (page 47)	Tex-Mex Bowl (page 77)	Broccoli-Parsnip Soup (page 50)	Kimchi Chicken Lettuce Cups (page 83)	Beet Gazpacho (page 36)
DINNER	Chickpea & Escarole Soup (page 51)	Zoodle Chow Mein (page 104)	Tex-Mex Bowl (page 77)	Peruvian Chicken Cauli Rice Soup (page 44)	Chicken & Zucchini Kefta (page 138)	Faux Meat Beet Tacos (page 100)	Chicken & Cabbage Dim Sum (page 145)

A FEW GO-TO SNACKS:

- Hard-boiled egg
- Handful of walnuts
- Toasted nori

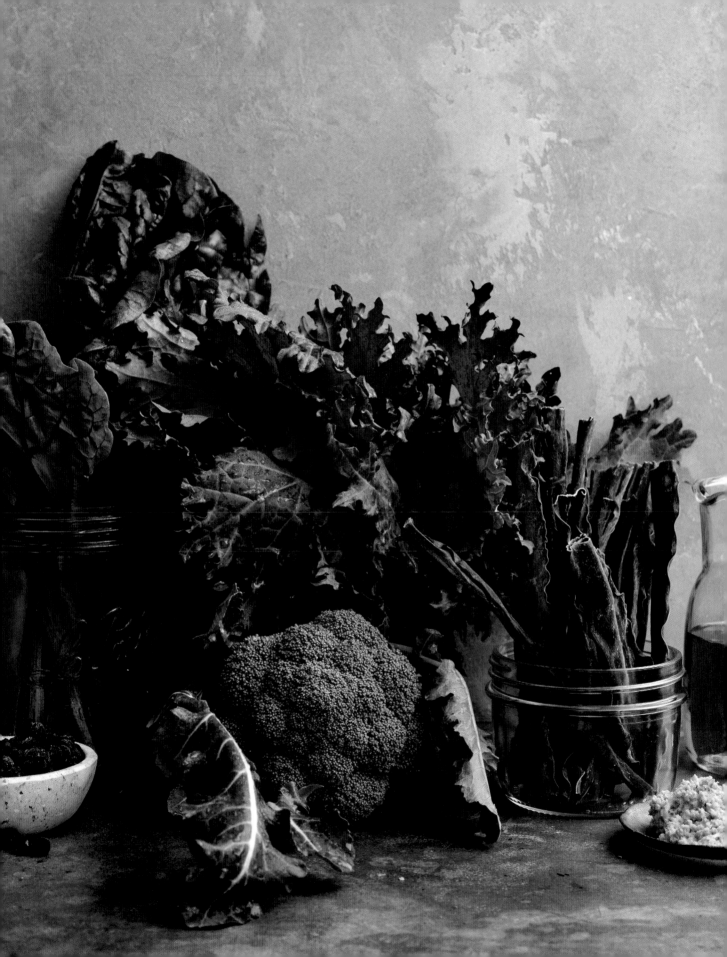

ADRENAL
SUPPORT

"Why am I so effing tired?" is a mantra widespread well beyond goop. The answer may be apparent in some instances (not enough rest, too much doing), but the effects on our bodies can be complex and sometimes masquerade as other health issues, explains LA-based cardiologist and functional medicine physician Alejandro Junger. A longtime friend and mentor of mine, Dr. Junger studies the phenomenon of adrenal fatigue (which is unrecognized by Western medicine). Junger likens the adrenals, the two small glands that sit on top of our kidneys and regulate the fight-or-flight reaction, to the power strip into which our organs are plugged for energy. When they are overworked (because of high stress and nonstop fight-or-flight reactions), we can feel tapped out. His tips for recharging follow.

A Q&A WITH ALEJANDRO JUNGER, MD

Q: Can you explain adrenal fatigue? What causes it?

A: To understand adrenal fatigue, first imagine this: You wake up early in the morning and have a good sweat working out. Then you prepare breakfast for the kids and take them to school. You go to work and have a busy day. Back to school to get the kids. Drive them around for their activities. Back home. Dinner. Bath and put them to sleep. You're exhausted—you can barely think or walk around. If at that very moment you went to the doctor and got a full physical and a set of blood tests, everything would be normal. But you know that everything is not "normal." You are exhausted. And the solution is so simple: a good night's sleep.

Like so many things in modern Western medicine that are not measurable and quantifiable, adrenal fatigue is rarely recognized (or even considered an issue). What Western medicine does recognize is the complete shutdown of the adrenal glands, called Addison's disease, and the other extreme, Cushing's disease, which presents as a hyperactive adrenal system. But I've seen a whole spectrum in the middle with patients. It's on the hypoactive side of the spectrum that we talk about adrenal fatigue.

The adrenal glands are small glands that sit on top of the kidneys, but their function in the body is anything but small. They are most famous for being responsible for creating the necessary inner conditions for a fight-or-flight response, which is a primitive way (physiologically speaking) of animals responding to danger, and therefore essential for survival. In natural conditions, the fight-or-flight response is activated only every now and then, depending on the surroundings. Between dangerous

moments, there is time to recover, then to just function at a baseline level. But modern life is very different from what nature designed. There are mini or major fight-or-flight responses triggered all day long, week after week, month after month, year after year. Anything that your mind interprets as threatening can get the adrenals firing adrenaline. In this constant state of stress, the adrenals must continuously attempt to adapt by releasing cortisol.

This chronic increase in adrenal activity can start taking a toll, as it would with any organ that is overused. Cortisol may be manufactured slower at times, faster at others, not following the normal circadian rhythm that allows for optimal functioning of the body. Instead of being released on awakening to help get us ready for a day of activities, cortisol may be low and slow early in the day. Instead of winding down at night to get the body ready for sleep, higher levels of cortisol may be released, making it difficult to get a good night's rest. This is one of the ways to indirectly "measure" a fatigued adrenal system—by testing cortisol levels, best done in saliva, at different times of the day and seeing the pattern.

Q: What are the primary symptoms?

A: The adrenal glands are involved in much more than just the fight-or-flight reactions. One could argue that directly or indirectly, they affect every cell in the body: They have an effect on the sex hormone system, on the way we absorb and assimilate minerals, on the way we process and utilize sugar, on the health of our blood vessels, and even on our mood and chain of thoughts. So when the adrenal system gets "fatigued," there are a lot of potential ways that imbalance or dysfunction may manifest in the body.

Some of the most typical symptoms are tiredness, mental fog, inability to get a good night's sleep and wake up rested, difficulty losing weight, hair loss, and irritability. But the picture may be much more complicated.

As adrenal function is connected with the sex hormones, adrenal fatigue may present as hormonal imbalances—irregular periods or no periods at all, infertility, lack of libido, difficulty gaining muscle mass, sugar cravings.

Because of the adrenal relationship with insulin, glucagon, and the intestines, adrenal fatigue can present as insulin resistance, diabetes, high blood pressure, and other symptoms related to the mismanagement of sugar by the cells.

Since adrenal function and mineral absorption are related, the fatigue can present as osteoporosis.

Because of the intimate relationship with the gut, adrenal fatigue can present as digestive issues, and potentially even depression, as the gut manufactures 90 percent of the serotonin in our body.

We could go system by system, organ by organ, examining ways in which fatigued adrenal glands may hinder optimal function elsewhere in the body. I see and hear from people every day who feel and know there is something wrong, but who cannot get an answer from a traditional medical test. If this sounds like you, your best bet is to find a functional medicine doctor who can take a holistic look at your symptoms and figure out if your adrenals may be fatigued.

Q: What are the indirect ways of testing for adrenal fatigue?

A: As mentioned, testing cortisol levels throughout the day can provide hints at how the adrenals are functioning. Low levels of DHEA also suggest

that the adrenals may be fatigued. A doctor who has experience with adrenal fatigue will do a full assessment to make sure it is not actually a different disease or issue being mimicked by adrenal fatigue. The best way, though, is often to see how you respond to the ways in which the adrenals can be "rested and recovered."

Q: What do you recommend for resetting the adrenals? What's possible in terms of rebalancing, and how long does it typically take?

A: Resting is essential. The adrenal system is perfectly designed to act in bursts when needed and then recover pretty fast as well. If we lived as nature designed us to, a good rest would be enough to rebalance. But with our stressful lifestyles, we are constantly activating the adrenal response, so it may take more time to recharge. Depending on the severity of the adrenal fatigue, it may take a few weeks to a few months, or even up to a couple of years in severe cases, to completely rebalance. The good news is that while full recovery may take longer than we'd like, people typically begin to feel some benefits almost immediately.

As with any health problem, when the root of it is uncovered and corrected, everything tends to correct itself, and health is restored. This is what the body is constantly trying to do. The problem with adrenal fatigue is that our identities are often wrapped up with the root cause of it (e.g., being busy, hardworking, always on the go) so it may be difficult to make the necessary lifestyle changes (e.g., resting more). We may think that if we slow down, our work will suffer or we won't be able to be there for our kids and their busy schedules, but there are health consequences when we never stop to recharge. (Also, if we made our kids' lives less busy from a young age, could we potentially prevent them from having to drastically change their lifestyle in the future to recover from adrenal fatigue?)

It's important to not only rest your body by decreasing muscular activity, but also to rest from the conditions in your life that are triggering a fight-or-flight response. For most people, sleeping more and sleeping better is a good start. There are entire books written about this subject; some of the tried-and-true tips are to avoid electronics prior to bedtime, try a warm bath or shower, don't eat immediately before bed, and make your room as dark as possible.

Relaxing more and having more fun is essential. Laughing, spending time with family and friends, and helping others can all be forms of medicine (cheesy, but true) that allow for adrenal recovery, or at least slow the excessive consumption of adrenaline and other adrenal stress hormones. Both yoga and meditation have been scientifically proven to benefit overall health in so many ways.

Sometimes it is necessary to make a drastic change and leave a toxic job, or a toxic relationship. Resting from a stressful life may also be more complicated, and involve learning new ways to respond to the same situations if they are impossible to change, at least for now.

Q: Which foods do you recommend eliminating from and adding to the diet?

A: Just as it is recommended to eliminate or reduce toxic exposures and situations, it is the same inside—and nothing affects us inside more intimately and powerfully than food. To allow the adrenals to recover, you should avoid all foods that make more digestive work for the body, that carry toxins (e.g., processed foods), or that trigger an allergy or sensitivity in some way (a food allergy can cause a small fight-or-flight reaction of sorts).

If you don't know which foods negatively affect you, a good place to start is avoiding any foods with chemicals and sticking to a basic elimination diet—no sugar, dairy, alcohol, coffee, or gluten.

Good foods to include are ones rich in nutrients and not hard to digest, like olive oil and avocados, coconut and coconut oil, apple cider vinegar, green veggies, bone broth, free-range meats if you eat animal products, nuts, fermented foods, and fruits like berries and açai.

Replacing some meals with supercharged smoothies is a good practice. This means less digestive work, but plenty of available nutrients to absorb. I like to add spirulina, Celtic salt, raw almond butter, E3 (marine algae), and bee pollen to my smoothies, no matter what else I put in them.

Q: Do you recommend supplements?

A: There are many supplements that can potentially help your adrenals recover, depending on your individual nutrient deficiencies and needs. In general, these include vitamins B, C, D; minerals such as selenium and magnesium; and fish oils (e.g., DHEA). But the royal family of adrenal helpers are the adaptogenic herbs—such as ashwagandha, rhodiola, holy basil, licorice—that help the body adapt to stress. Moringa (from the moringa tree) can be another helpful adaptogen and contains most micronutrients needed for optimal body physiology; it can be taken as pills or in powder form (added to smoothies).

The Food Shortlist

BEST TO AVOID

- Alcohol
- Coffee
- Dairy
- Gluten
- Processed foods

- Red meat and shellfish
- Strawberries, bananas, grapefruit, and oranges
- Sugar

GOOD TO ADD

- Açai
- Apple cider vinegar
- Avocados
- Berries
- Fermented foods

- Green veggies
- Olive oil
- Seaweed

The goopified Menu

	MONDAY	TUESDAY	WEDNESDAY	THURSDAY	FRIDAY	SATURDAY	SUNDAY
BREAKFAST	Black Rice Pudding with Coconut Milk & Mango (page 27)	Blueberry Cauliflower Smoothie (page 164)	Quinoa Cereal with Freeze-Dried Berries (page 24)	Chocolate Chia Pudding (page 28)	Beet Açai Blueberry Smoothie Bowl (page 29)	Sweet Buckwheat Porridge (page 25)	Chlorella Smoothie (page 166)
LUNCH	Nori Salad Roll (page 93)	Beet Gazpacho (page 36)	Quinoa, Sweet Potato & Tahini Grain Bowl (page 68)	Grilled Chicken Salad with Miso Dressing (page 55)	Curry Chicken Lettuce Cups (page 84)	Garden Salad with Aquafaba Ranch Dressing (page 59)	Crunchy Spring Veggie Grain Bowl (page 66)
DINNER	Faux Meat Beet Tacos (page 100)	Kimchi Lettuce Cups (page 83)	Halibut en Papillote with Lemon, Mushrooms & Toasted Sesame Oil (page 114)	Braised Chicken Tacos on Butternut Squash "Tortillas" (page 103)	Teriyaki Bowl (page 73)	Herby Meatballs with Nomato Sauce (page 134)	Turkey Burgers (page 129)

A FEW GO-TO SNACKS:

- Toasted nori
- Seed Cracker (page 203) with avocado
- Handful of blueberries

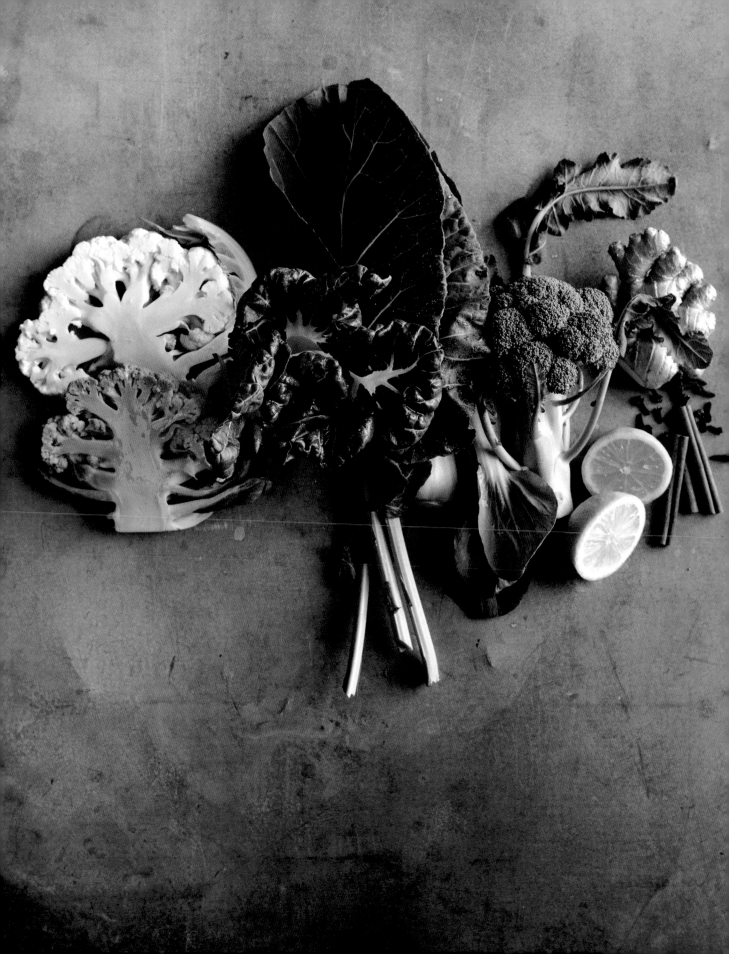

CANDIDA
RESET

Functional medicine expert Dr. Amy Myers (author of *The Autoimmune Solution* and *The Thyroid Connection*) has become an indispensable resource on women's health issues that are oft misunderstood, from thyroid dysfunction to gut imbalances like SIBO (small intestinal bacterial overgrowth). One of her specialties is helping people heal from an overgrowth of Candida, which is a form of yeast. Myers's primer on yeast overgrowth and how it might subtly affect the body (e.g., fatigue, bloating, eczema) is regularly referenced on goop.com, and many have leaned on her online Candida Breakthrough Program. A lot of her work and theories around health are based on her clinical experience and you won't necessarily see them reflected in classic scientific literature, or at least not yet. Her most recent book, *The Autoimmunity Cookbook*, is full of recipes designed to bring balance back to the gut. (Note: If you already follow Dr. Myers's self-designed protocols, you'll know that they are typically grain- and legume-free. She primarily works with patients who have autoimmunity and has found cutting out these foods to be helpful for them.)

A Q&A WITH AMY MYERS, MD

Q: What is Candida—where does it live in the body, and how does it differ from other fungal and yeast infections?

A: Candida is a fungus. A lot of people use the terms "yeast overgrowth" and "Candida" interchangeably, and there are hundreds of different types of yeast, but the most common form of yeast infection is known as *Candida albicans*.

Candida lives throughout our bodies in small amounts: in the oral cavity, digestive tract, gut microbiome, and vaginal tract. Its job is to aid with digestion and nutrient absorption—which it does when it's in balance with the good bacteria in your microbiome. I think of the microbiome (clusters of mainly bacteria, plus other organisms, found in our skin, nose, mouth, gut, urinary tract) as a rain forest: When everything is in balance, the body is in harmony and runs smoothly.

Problems occur when there is too much Candida in relation to your body's good bacteria, and it overpowers the bacteria, which can lead to leaky gut and a host of other digestive issues, as well as fungal infections, mood swings, and brain fog. (Leaky gut is when the junctions in the intestinal lining break apart, and particles including toxins escape from your intestines and travel throughout your body via your bloodstream.) People generally equate Candida with a systemic overgrowth—e.g., a vaginal yeast infection in a woman, or a nail fungus. But the signs of Candida overgrowth can be subtler. Conventional medicine only recognizes the systemic and often fatal form of Candida overgrowth known as candidemia, which is when Candida invades the blood. About 90 percent of the patients I see (people who are sick, have autoimmune disorders, leaky gut, etc.) have

Candida overgrowth that, while not fatal, is extremely disruptive to their health. Like, say, adrenal fatigue, which also has pervasive, seemingly vague symptoms, this level of Candida overgrowth is not really recognized by conventional medicine.

The symptoms of different kinds of yeast infections overlap greatly (although some lead to infections in different parts of the body), and the vast majority of treatment is the same. Lab work can distinguish which type of yeast infection you have.

Q: What causes an overgrowth of Candida?

A: There are a number of factors that can contribute to Candida—the major ones are:

Diet: A diet high in sugar, refined carbohydrates, and processed foods makes it easy for yeast to multiply and thrive—these are the foods yeast lives off of. Alcohol, which tends to involve a lot of yeast, sugar, and carbs (e.g., beer and wine), is also problematic.

Antibiotics & Other Medications: Taking even one round of antibiotics can kill too much of your body's good bacteria and throw off the balance of your microbiome. A mom's microbiome also affects her baby's developing microbiome—so if a mother takes antibiotics while pregnant, or had yeast infections, that can contribute to yeast overgrowth in the child. As can C-sections, which affect a baby's microbiome. Steroids can also cause a yeast overgrowth, as can acid-blocking pills (you need enough acid to kill bacteria and parasites on your food, some yeasts, as well as viruses).

Oral Contraceptives: Yeast likes high-estrogen conditions, so we see a correlation between birth control use and yeast overgrowth.

Stress: A high-stress lifestyle may also lead Candida to overpower the good bacteria in your microbiome.

Q: What symptoms are typically associated with Candida overgrowth?

A: When the body overproduces Candida, it may break down the wall of the intestine, causing leaky gut and releasing toxic by-products into your body. Leaky gut disrupts your body's ability to digest and absorb nutrients (causing nutrition deficiencies), and can lead to health issues beyond digestive concerns, including autoimmunity and thyroid dysfunction.

In addition to leaky gut, the other overarching problem associated with Candida is a suppressed immune system. About 60 to 80 percent of our immune system lives in our gut. Yeast overgrowth is associated with a suppressed production of IgA—the antibody immunoglobulin A, which is vital to immunity. Most of the patients I see with Candida overgrowth also suffer immunity issues.

The common signs of Candida overgrowth are:

- Brain fog, poor memory, ADHD
- Fatigue and/or fibromyalgia
- Autoimmune diseases connected to leaky gut (as mentioned above)
- Digestive issues—gas, bloating, constipation
- Skin issues, including eczema, hives, rosacea, rashes
- Seasonal allergies/chronic sinus infections
- Skin and nail fungal infections (ringworm, athlete's foot, tinea versicolor—when you get white spots in the sun): An external fungus can be an isolated issue, but is often a sign that the rest of the body is imbalanced.

- Vaginal infections, UTIs
- Sugar cravings: Sugar is food for yeast.
- Mercury overload: Some alternative medicine experts think yeast overgrowths can manifest to surround and protect mercury in the body.

Q: How do you test for Candida?

A: The tests I use to diagnose Candida are:

Antibodies: I check for total IgG, IgM, and IgA antibodies to see if your immune system is mounting a response to an infection—i.e., if your levels are high. A low level of IgA, however, could indicate that you have a suppressed immune system and that your body is not able to mount a response. I also check for IgG, IgA, and IgM Candida antibodies in your blood—high levels of these antibodies may indicate that you have a Candida overgrowth that your immune system is responding to. (Any lab can order these blood tests.)

Complete Blood Count (CBC): A low white blood cell count (WBC) has been associated with yeast overgrowth, as well as a high neutrophil and low lymphocyte count. Although not specific to yeast, I see this pattern frequently in patients with Candida overgrowth.

Stool Test: You'll need to seek out a functional medicine doctor and ask for a comprehensive (rather than standard) stool test, which will include a check for Candida in your colon/large intestines. (It will also check your level of IgA in stool.) From a stool test, the lab can usually identify the type of yeast (if it is not Candida) and the most effective treatment path.

Organix Dysbiosis Urine Test: This test looks at a marker of the Candida waste product (like anything, yeast excretes waste) called D-arabinitol. A high level may indicate that there is yeast overgrowth in the upper gut/small intestines.

Infection: A swab of a yeast infection can be sent off to the lab for analysis to determine which type of yeast you have.

There is a self-spit test (find it with a simple Google search)—which doesn't have a lot of scientific data around it—that I know many of my patients have done on their own before coming into the office. Most of the time, I find that the other tests I do confirm that the patient has an overgrowth, but again, the spit test is not as exact as these medical tests.

Q: What's the best treatment plan?

A: The best way to treat Candida is with a three-step approach:

1. STARVE THE YEAST

The first step is to eliminate foods that have yeast in them and foods that yeast likes to eat.

This means cutting out vinegar, beer, wine, mushrooms (as part of the fungi family, they can cross-react with Candida), sugar, refined carbs, and processed foods.

But you also want to limit healthy carbs like legumes, grains, and starchy veggies to 1 cup a day, and fruit to a single piece a day—because, unfortunately, even good carbs feed yeast.

Along the same lines, I tell people to hold off on good fermented foods (not something all doctors agree on)—e.g., sauerkraut, pickles, kimchi—until they've killed off the yeast. While these foods are beneficial for the good bacteria in your microbiome, they also are good for yeast (which isn't helpful if you have an overgrowth).

2. OVERPOWER THE YEAST

Some patients need a prescription antifungal (like Diflucan or Nystatin).

Antifungal supplements can be effective, too: My two go-to supplements are caprylic acid (naturally found in coconut oil) and Candifense (which contains enzymes that break down parasitic and fungal cell walls). Some people take oil of oregano, which is broad spectrum, meaning that it will kill good and bad organisms in the microbiome, but I try to stick with more targeted supplements that really only kill yeast.

3. REPLENISH GOOD BACTERIA

During treatment, take high-quality probiotic supplements, which help protect your body against future infections. You don't want to take prebiotics—which feed good bacteria and yeast—while you're trying to get rid of Candida, but you can add them in, along with fermented foods, down the line once your Candida is under control.

Q: Are there ways to get rid of Candida without going on such a restrictive diet? Are there beneficial foods you can add to your diet to combat Candida?

A: It's really hard to get rid of Candida without adjusting your diet—even if you're on an antifungal prescription, you need to take away the foods that are contributing to the overgrowth.

Foods you want to add to your diet are:

Coconut Oil: Contains caprylic acid (mentioned above), which kills yeast cells.

Olive Oil: The antioxidants in olive oil help your body get rid of Candida.

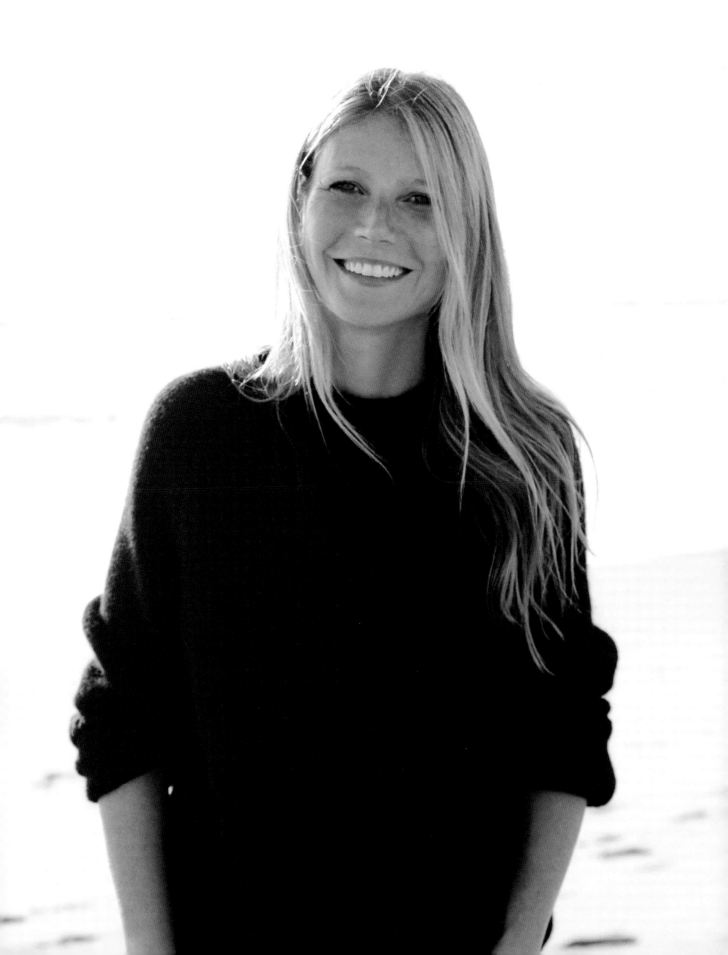

Garlic: Contains allicin, a sulfur-containing compound with specific-to-Candida antifungal properties.

Cinnamon: Has antifungal and anti-inflammatory benefits.

Apple Cider Vinegar: This is the only vinegar I recommend consuming while you're treating a Candida overgrowth—its enzymes may help break down Candida.

Lemon: Has some antifungal properties, and helps your liver detox.

Ginger: Has anti-inflammatory and antifungal properties—plus, it supports your liver.

Cloves: Very effective (internal) antifungal. Clove oil can also be used as a topical aid for infections.

Cruciferous Veggies: Broccoli, radishes, Brussels sprouts, cabbage, etc., have sulfur- and nitrogen-containing compounds that attack Candida.

Wild Salmon: Omega-3 fatty acids help fight fungal infections.

Q: How long does it typically take to get rid of a Candida overgrowth?

A: It largely depends on what caused the Candida overgrowth. Let's say it was a one-off scenario: You had bronchitis, went through two rounds of antibiotics, and got Candida. After a few weeks of a Candida cleanse (i.e., following the diet guidelines here), you can likely get rid of the overgrowth, restore your gut microbiome, and move on. I have a thirty-day program online at amymyersmd.com that can get you started.

If it wasn't a one-off situation, it likely won't be a quick fix. While this doesn't mean that you can't ever have a glass of wine or a slice of cake again, you might find that you feel your best with longer-term adjustments to your diet.

The Food Shortlist

BEST TO AVOID

- Beer and wine
- Fermented foods
- Healthy carbs like legumes, grains, and starchy veggies (limit to 1 cup a day) and fruit (limit to 1 piece a day)
- Mushrooms
- Sugar, refined carbs, processed foods
- Vinegar (except apple cider vinegar)

GOOD TO ADD

- Apple cider vinegar
- Cinnamon
- Cloves
- Coconut oil
- Cruciferous vegetables
- Garlic
- Ginger
- Lemons
- Olive oil
- Wild salmon

The goopified Menu

	MONDAY	TUESDAY	WEDNESDAY	THURSDAY	FRIDAY	SATURDAY	SUNDAY
BREAKFAST	Strawberry Cauliflower Smoothie (page 163)	Seed Cracker with Smoked Salmon & Avocado (page 15)	Blueberry Cauliflower Smoothie (page 164)	Zucchini & Lemon Soccata (page 10)	Seed Cracker with Egg & Avocado (page 16)	Sweet Buckwheat Porridge (page 25)	Kale Kuku Soccata (page 8)
LUNCH	Tarragon Chicken Lettuce Cups (page 86)	Kale, Carrot & Avo Salad with Tahini Dressing (page 63)	Crunchy Summer Rolls (page 91)	Roasted Kabocha Soup (page 35)	Brown Rice Grain Bowl with Kale, Broccoli & Sesame (page 65)	Cucumber & Avocado Gazpacho (page 40)	Grilled Chicken Salad with Miso Dressing (page 55)
DINNER	Coconut Chicken Soup (page 41)	Black Rice with Braised Chicken Thighs (page 109)	Five-Spice Salmon Burgers (page 125)	Sheet Pan Chicken with Broccolini & Radicchio (page 120)	Chickpea & Kale Curry (page 141)	Beet Falafel Sliders (page 123)	Italian Braised Chicken (page 130)

A FEW GO-TO SNACKS:

- Raw broccoli and cauliflower with Aquafaba Ranch Dressing (page 181)
- Hot water with ginger and lemon
- Half an avocado with lemon, sea salt, grated fresh ginger, and toasted sesame oil

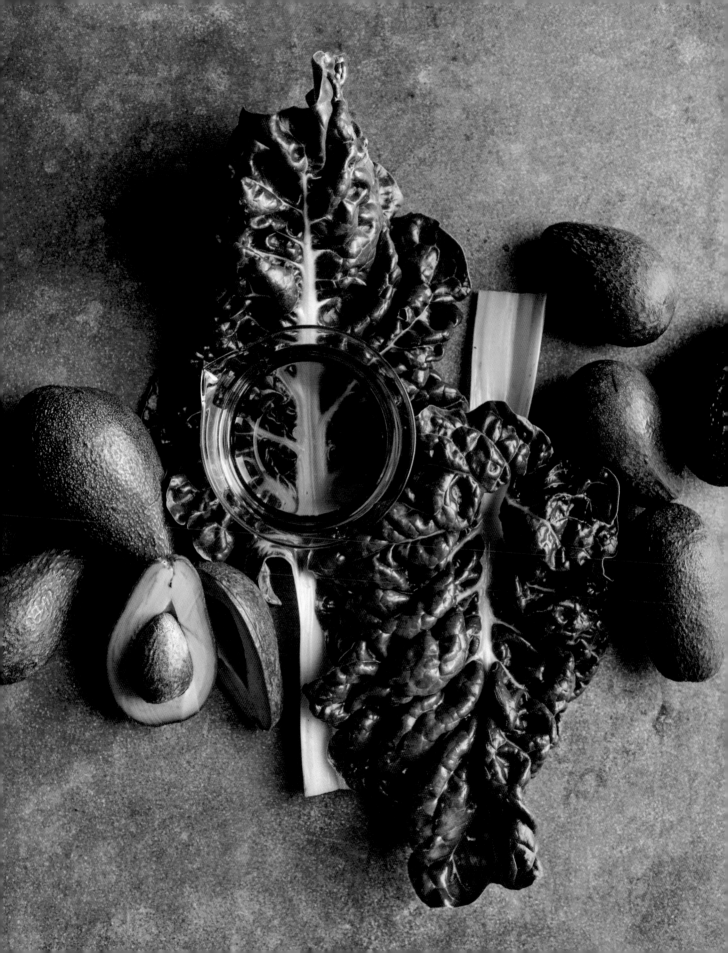

HEART HEALTH

"If I ate bread at every meal, for every day of my life, I'd be a happy but miserable guy," Dr. Steven Gundry begins our conversation on his food philosophy. Gundry, a cardiologist by training, served as chairman and head of cardiothoracic surgery at Loma Linda University School of Medicine for sixteen years. In 2001, he met a so-called hopeless patient with heart disease who ended up turning around his health by making some surprising diet adjustments. This experience changed the trajectory of Dr. Gundry's career, who went on to explore the power of nutrition, and search for cures for notoriously difficult-to-treat diseases and disorders. As the founder and director of the Center for Restorative Medicine, based in Palm Springs, California, he's helped his patients to reverse significant cardiovascular damage—in part by removing lectins, a plant-based protein, from their diet. For much more on his dietary research, see his books *The Plant Paradox*, *The Plant Paradox Cookbook*, and *Dr. Gundry's Diet Evolution*.

A Q&A WITH
STEVEN GUNDRY, MD

Q: What's the greatest cardiovascular health concern?

A: Heart disease, in both men and women, is the number one killer in the United States. While there's certainly no need for fearmongering, we should look at it seriously. Women's complaints around their heart and chest are not always taken seriously enough. Women often don't have the same symptoms that we teach men about heart disease, such as the feeling of an elephant sitting on the chest, or pain going down the left arm or into the jaw. With women, signs of heart disease, coronary artery disease, narrowing in the arteries, can be as simple as fatigue, or shortness of breath, or nausea, or feeling sick after meals. Women should be empowered to take their health concerns seriously, and as doctors, we can't just dismiss these symptoms as "female complaints," because too many women are not getting the care they should.

Q: Which risk factors should people be proactively aware of?

A: Cholesterol levels in general don't have a lot to do with developing heart disease. Around half the people who present to the ER with chest pain or a heart attack have normal levels of LDL, the so-called bad cholesterol. But there is one genetic risk related to a type of cholesterol that most people are unaware of: It's an inherited gene that tells the body to make the cholesterol lipoprotein(a), or Lp(a). The gene is very common in northern Europeans, the English, Irish, and Scottish; and is typically present in families with strong histories of heart disease. I ask everyone to have their doctor measure their Lp(a) levels, which is an $8 test. While statin drugs are generally not effective if you have this gene, it turns out that taking niacin (a form of vitamin B$_3$) is extremely beneficial.

Triglycerides (a type of fat in the blood) are one of the biggest mischief makers contributing to heart disease. The body converts calories it doesn't need immediately into triglycerides, to be used for energy later. When we overeat sugar (even in the form of fruit), we make excess triglycerides. One of the best predictors for *avoiding* heart disease is to have HDL ("good cholesterol") levels that are higher than your triglyceride levels. I've read several papers that suggest that cutting back on sugars, including natural sugars found in fruit and seeded vegetables, can help improve the ratio of HDL to triglycerides.

Q: What's possible when it comes to reversing damage already done to the heart?

A: At our clinic, we help people reverse severe blockages in their coronary arteries largely through diet and lifestyle changes. We've collected data from ten thousand patients who we have followed for fifteen years. Every three months, we use a number of sophisticated blood tests (that Medicare and insurance generally pay for) to test how well patients are doing. When people follow the protocol, we see their good cholesterol go up and their bad cholesterol go down. But, most important, we see the amount of inflammation on the inside of their blood vessels decrease, or even completely resolve itself.

Q: Can you explain the food philosophy behind your cardiovascular-focused program?

A: One of the principles of the program is to lessen the amount of lectin-containing foods that people eat. Lectins are proteins found in certain plants that are meant to protect the plants from predators. Lectins are sometimes called sticky proteins, because they seek out particular sugar molecules on cells in our blood, the lining of our gut, and on our nerves. Lectins can prompt attacks on the lining of our blood vessels, too. While some people seem to react more vigorously to lectins than others, we've found that eliminating them from the diet helps to reverse cardiovascular blockages across our patient group. We've also seen markers of inflammation go up again when lectin-heavy foods have been reintroduced to our patients' diet.

The main lectin-containing foods are grains, seeded vegetables/fruits like nightshades and squashes, and legumes. In plants, the lectins are found in the peels and seeds, so you can get rid of them by, for instance, peeling and seeding tomatoes before making sauce (which is how Italians have traditionally cooked). Pressure cooking beans, tomatoes, potatoes, and grains is also an effective way to get rid of the lectins before you eat these foods. (Note that this doesn't work for wheat, oats, rye, barley, or spelt.)

In general, fruits and seeded vegetables—which are technically fruits—should have a limited place in a heart-healthy diet. Our modern fruits have been bred for sugar content, and while we now have fruit 365 days a year, just 50 years ago, our fruit consumption was seasonal.

I have no issues with colleagues who say that some of the healthiest people in the world traditionally eat grain and beans, but people who follow that diet in these longevity hot spots tend to have vastly different immune systems than the average American. They also haven't been exposed to our lifestyle, the toxins in our environment, the number of antibiotics we take, the amount of antibiotics fed to the animals we eat, anti-inflammatory drugs like Advil and Aleve that can damage the gut lining, pesticides like glyphosate that change our gut bacteria, and so on.

I do believe, though, that we can learn and adopt other habits from the world's healthiest people. For example, I think a secret of extreme longevity is limiting animal protein so that it is more of a garnishment, or flavoring, and not the main focus of every meal.

Q: Which foods should we be eating more of?

A: One of my favorite sayings is that the only purpose of food is to get olive oil into your mouth. Several of the world's longest-lived populations use a liter of olive oil per week. The only reasonable way to eat close to that much olive oil is to pour it on your food. Think of broccoli, or a couple of poached eggs, or a piece of fish, as a delivery device for olive oil. Whatever you're eating, bring your olive oil to the table, too.

Q: Can any supplements make a difference in cardiovascular health?

A: We have a big vitamin D deficiency in this country. For my average patient, I recommend taking 5,000 IU/day. Vitamin E is essential for heart health. Fish oil, particularly the DHA component, is important for overall health and for keeping the gut wall intact.

Polyphenols are plant compounds that are primarily found in dark fruit and dark leafy greens. They interact with gut bacteria and are turned into compounds that have been shown to make our blood vessels more flexible and make the inside lining of the blood vessels slippery. Which is a good thing. Cholesterol is not interested in your blood vessel lining unless there's inflammation or "stickiness" on the wall. We've found that after introducing polyphenols into people's diet, the stickiness goes away. (If they stop taking polyphenols, that stickiness comes back.) Common polyphenols include grapeseed extract, green tea, black coffee, and cacao (dark chocolate is good for this reason). I make a polyphenol-based product called Vital Reds, but you can get grapeseed extract nearly anywhere, including at Costco.

Q: What about exercise, stress, and other lifestyle factors?

A: Exercise definitely has a place in heart health. I try to have my patients spend less time working on aerobic exercises like running and more time on strength training like yoga and Pilates. You can think of it this way: Our muscles are the customers that buy sugars from a hormone called insulin. The more muscle mass you carry, and the hungrier muscles are, the easier it is to get sugar out of the bloodstream. Chronically elevated insulin, or prediabetes, is prevalent in the vast majority of people who have heart disease, so you want your insulin level to be as normal or low as possible.

The old idea that chronic stress—like what you might expect someone with a type A personality to experience—causes heart disease has pretty much gone by the wayside. I don't typically see stress having a significant effect on heart disease.

Q: Why do you recommend fasting? Who is it not for?

A: We are realizing that a twenty-four-hour period of fasting may have the potential to reset the message in our stem cells in the lining of our gut, of all things, to begin to grow and divide. All you might need is a twenty-four-hour period of time without eating to really reset the stem cells in your gut, which, in simplistic terms, helps heal the gut. I believe that almost all chronic disease is the result of gut issues, and that longevity begins in the gut. A lot of ancient wisdom recognized the importance of fasting in optimal health and almost every great religious group practiced a period of fasting.

For a full-on fast, you just drink water for twenty-four hours; most people don't really need anything else but consult your doctor around any health concerns. People who do poorly with fasting, in general, have high-insulin levels. People who are prediabetic or diabetic can't use fat stores to fuel their brain. I have these patients take MCT oil or coconut oil during that fasting period. Pregnant mothers should not fast.

The Food Shortlist

BEST TO AVOID

- Grains (sorghum and millet are okay because they don't have a hull and thus don't contain lectins)

- Polyunsaturated oils like canola and corn, safflower oil

- Seeded vegetables/fruits (okay if you seed and peel)

  Note: Pressure cook your legumes (or buy them already pressure cooked from the brand Eden Foods) to get rid of the lectins first.

GOOD TO ADD

- Avocado
- Cruciferous vegetables
- Leafy greens
- Olive oil
- Turmeric

The goopified Menu

	MONDAY	TUESDAY	WEDNESDAY	THURSDAY	FRIDAY	SATURDAY	SUNDAY
BREAKFAST	Easy Frittata (page 21)	Blueberry Cauliflower Smoothie (page 164)	Beet Açai Blueberry Smoothie Bowl (page 29)	Fast	Poached Eggs over Sautéed Greens (page 22)	Veggie Scramble (page 19)	Blueberry Cauliflower Smoothie (page 164)
LUNCH	Chicken Larb Lettuce Cups (page 87)	Clean Carrot Soup (page 33)	Italian Chicken Salad with Grilled Asparagus (page 58)	Fast	Kimchi Chicken Lettuce Cups (page 83)	Kale & Sweet Potato Salad with Miso (page 80)	Cucumber & Avocado Gazpacho (page 40)
DINNER	Fish Tacos on Jicama "Tortillas" (page 99)	Chicken & Cabbage Dim Sum (page 145)	Halibut en Papillote with Lemon, Mushrooms & Toasted Sesame Oil (page 114)	Fast	Za'atar Chicken Bowl (page 74)	Za'atar Chicken Bowl (page 74)	Sheet Pan Chicken Curry (page 119)

A FEW GO-TO SNACKS:

- Hot water with lemon

- Cucumber (peeled and seeded) and avocado with lime and salt

- Hard-boiled egg

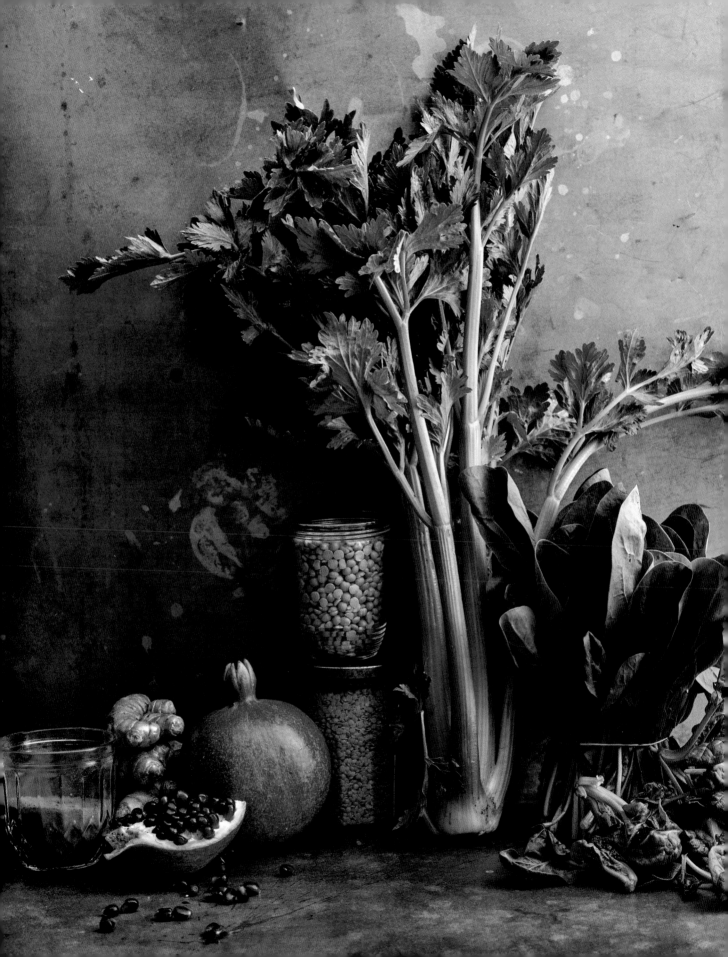

VEG-FRIENDLY AYURVEDA

There are seemingly few nutritional tenets that everyone agrees on but most health experts I talk to lean into plant-heavy diets. Of course, this isn't just a modern trend—some of the most well-known vegetable-centric cleanses stem from ancient Ayurveda.

An expert in Ayurvedic and holistic health, Aruna Viswanathan is the head of the ear, nose, and throat department and integrative medicine director at Vikram Hospital and Research Institute in Coimbatore, India. She lives in Goa, where she currently practices out of a center called the Renewal Point. As the medical advisor of the brand ORGANIC INDIA, Viswanathan is adept at making Ayurvedic principles of cleansing approachable and accessible to the novice.

A Q&A WITH
ARUNA VISWANATHAN,
MBBS, MS (ENT), FAGE

Q: Who can benefit from an Ayurvedic cleanse? What kind of results do people typically feel/see, and at what point?

A: Anyone who wants to be well or healthier; almost everyone is a candidate with the exception of children, pregnant/nursing mothers, and those with conflicting health conditions. Benefits often include: improved energy, digestion, skin and hair health. Most people report "glowing" or "shining" after an Ayurvedic cleanse. Sugar and food cravings may go away as early as the first or second week.

The typical cleanse is twenty-one days because we generally need at least three weeks to form lifelong healthy habits that can truly be a gateway to a new life of radiant health. But people usually see results in even just one week, feeling lighter as energy levels rise. (A lot of people are amazed that they don't need more food to feel so energized.) Mental clarity and increased energy are tangible for the first time.

After a twenty-one-day cleanse, each week, you can reintroduce a new food group to your diet, and really experience how it affects you, as your body will be like a "clean slate." This knowledge, and being able to understand your own body, is another benefit of the cleanse.

Q: What do people typically eat (and not eat) during an Ayurvedic cleanse?

A: An Ayurvedic protocol consists of ancient cleansing herbs that support detoxification and nutritionally complete meals.

The diet is rich in beans, greens, and other vegetables (all organic). Celery, parsley, cilantro, amaranth, and spinach are all known as cleansing vegetables. All lentils and legumes may be used, unless you have trouble digesting them (for instance, chickpeas can be difficult for some to digest).

It's also important to drink plenty of water.

Local, organic, seasonal fruits are preferred. Lemons, grapefruits, and limes can all aid in cleansing. Astringent fruits like pomegranate, cranberries, and jamun (a type of plum) are also beneficial. Certain sweet fruits (like persimmons and grapes) and packaged fruit juices should be avoided.

The main ingredients to avoid are animal products (including seafood), white sugar, refined white flour, and dairy. These ingredients are known as "clogging foods" in Ayurveda, and do not support cleansing.

Preferably also avoid bread made with yeast and nightshades (known as energetically blocking in Ayurveda), including potatoes (which can be difficult to digest). Mushrooms should not be eaten often.

You can follow the individual foods that are recommended/discouraged for your particular *dosha*—there are three mind-body types or energies. But cleansing is vital irrespective of *dosha*, and set

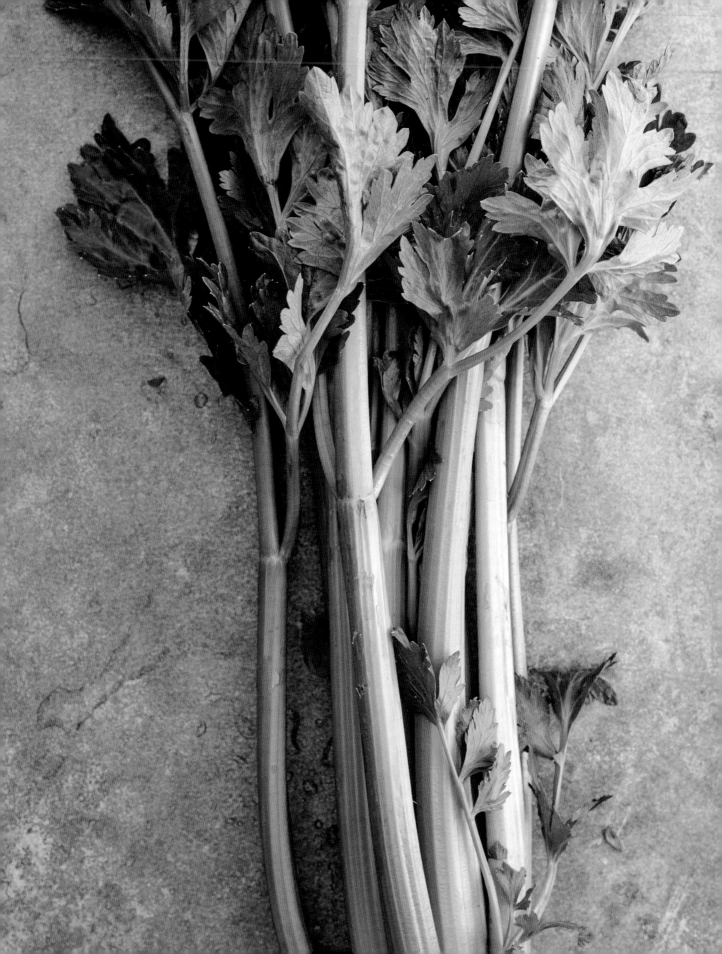

Ayurvedic cleanses like ORGANIC INDIA's REVIVE kit can be used by people of all *doshas*. (ORGANIC INDIA's kit is a collaborative creation by many experts across the world, and the most friendly way I know of to do an Ayurvedic cleanse at home. It includes complete protein, fiber, superfoods, greens, and probiotics that are instrumental in nourishment and detoxification.)

Q: What are some of the best foods and herbs?

A: Kitchari (also spelled khichri or khichdi), a combination of steamed beans and rice sautéed with ghee and cumin seeds, is a staple of Ayurvedic detoxes. *Moong dal khichri* is made with mung beans—considered the lightest of all legumes and *sattvic* food. In Ayurveda, *sattvic* foods are fresh, whole, nutrient dense, and high in prana (meaning vital energy), as they are cooked with love. They are meant to balance all the elements and nourish consciousness, mind, and body.

Kanji, or rice porridge, can be made with gluten-free grains like millet, buckwheat, or brown, white, black, or wild rice. Cassava flour is very light and great for cooking during a detox. While dairy should be avoided, ghee is great, but should be organic A2 cow ghee.

Amla is the best fruit, along with *haritaki* and *bibhitaki*. These fruits are not easy to source fresh in most parts of the world but are available together as capsules or in powder form called triphala from ORGANIC INDIA and others. I describe triphala as a gentle, effective scrub for the insides, designed to support the health of the GI tract, digestion, and elimination. It contains vitamin C and other antioxidants, promotes good health, and has long been used to balance all three *doshas*. I use triphala extensively in my practice and recommend it with warm water when you wake up and before bed (not with food).

Other important herbs include tulsi (holy basil), *bhumyamalaki*, neem, and *punarnava*, which are part of the ORGANIC INDIA REVIVE kit. The precise combination of herbs have been specially formulated to enhance the cleansing process in the comfort of your own home, but it's always best to consult a physician, particularly if you have any specific health issues.

Q: Are there any other important guidelines?

- As mentioned, stay well hydrated. Warm water and water with lemon can help flush toxins out. But avoid drinking water during meals and right after eating, as this can impair digestion and "kill the digestive fire."
- All food that reduces *ama*, or toxic buildup, is great during a cleanse. Old food from the refrigerator increases *ama*, and you also want to steer clear of fried, greasy, and heavy food during cleansing.
- The prana (energy) of food is highest when eaten in the first 3-4 hours after preparing it.
- Eat your biggest meal at noon, when the sun is up, as that is when the *agni*, or digestive fire, is at its peak.
- Avoid fruits and salads in the evening, as they aren't digested quickly.
- Spend an hour in the sun and stand barefoot on the earth for a few minutes every day, if you can.

Q: What do you suggest beyond diet and supplementation?

A: Exercise, meditation—and fun—are integral parts of cleansing. Exercise until you break into a sweat and then shower right after to help your body remove toxins. Oil pulling and dry brushing are also bonus techniques used to enhance cleansing and detoxification.

The Food Shortlist

BEST TO AVOID

- Dairy (ghee is okay)
- Eggs
- Gluten
- Meat, poultry, and seafood
- Nightshades
- Refined sugar (a little stevia, monk fruit, or honey is okay)

GOOD TO ADD

- Celery
- Cilantro
- Ginger
- Lemons, grapefruits, and limes
- Lentils
- Parsley
- Pomegranate
- Rice
- Spinach
- Turmeric

The goopified Menu

	MONDAY	TUESDAY	WEDNESDAY	THURSDAY	FRIDAY	SATURDAY	SUNDAY
BREAKFAST	Beet Açai Blueberry Smoothie Bowl (page 29)	Quinoa Cereal with Freeze-Dried Berries (page 24)	Sweet Buckwheat Porridge (page 25)	Breakfast Dal (page 11)	Black Rice Pudding with Coconut Milk & Mango (page 27)	Chlorella Smoothie (page 166)	Chocolate Chia Pudding (page 28)
LUNCH	Crunchy Summer Rolls (page 91)	Miso Soup (page 47)	Kitchari (page 110)	Crunchy Spring Veggie Grain Bowl (page 66)	Clean Carrot Soup (page 33)	Garden Salad with Aquafaba Ranch Dressing (page 59)	Kale & Sweet Potato Salad with Miso (page 80)
DINNER	Brown Rice, Turmeric & Spinach Porridge (page 48)	White Bean & Zucchini Burgers (page 124)	Kale Aglio e Olio (page 133)	Faux Meat Beet Tacos (page 100)	Chickpea & Kale Curry (page 141)	Broccoli-Parsnip Soup (page 50)	Beet Falafel Sliders (page 123)

A FEW GO-TO SNACKS:

- Hot water with ginger, lemon, and turmeric
- Handful of pomegranate seeds
- Brown rice with furikake
- Half a grapefruit

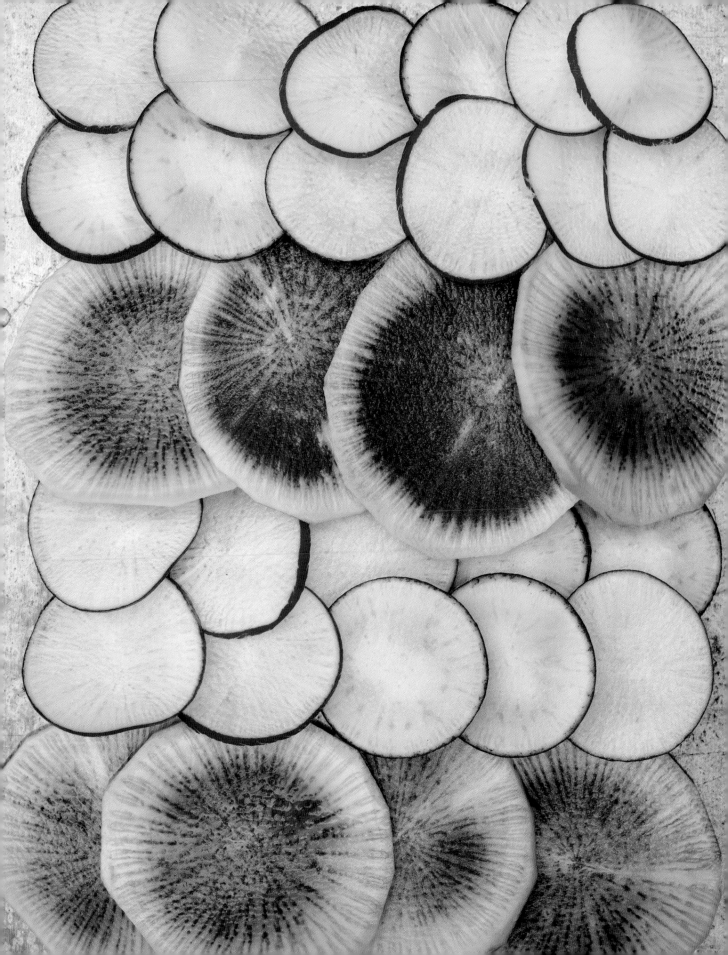

ACKNOWLEDGMENTS

TEAM GOOP

Thea Baumann
Ana Hito
Kevin Keating
Kiki Koroshetz

Elise Loehnen
Kelly Martin
Caitlin O'Malley

PHOTOGRAPHER

Ditte Isager

ASSISTED BY:
Graham Dalton
Conner Hughes
Rasmus Jensen

PROP STYLIST

Kate Martindale

ASSISTED BY:
Ian Hartman
Ali Summers

FOOD STYLIST

Susie Theodorou

ASSISTED BY:
Thea Baumann
Ana Hito

CLOTHING STYLIST

Ali Pew

ASSISTED BY:
Amy Wilbraham

PRODUCER

Kendall Stewart

ASSISTED BY:
Jacob Arzola
Ross Gardner
Vinnie Maggio
Alex Rubenstein

ART DIRECTION AND DESIGN

Michelle Park

Shubhani Sarkar

GRAND CENTRAL LIFE & STYLE

Jimmy Franco
Morgan Hedden
Brittany McInerney

Karen Murgolo
Amanda Pritzker
Kallie Shimek

THANKS, TOO

Terry Abbott
Jeffery Mahlick
Victoria Ortiz

Veronica Rivera
Maria Rosales

257

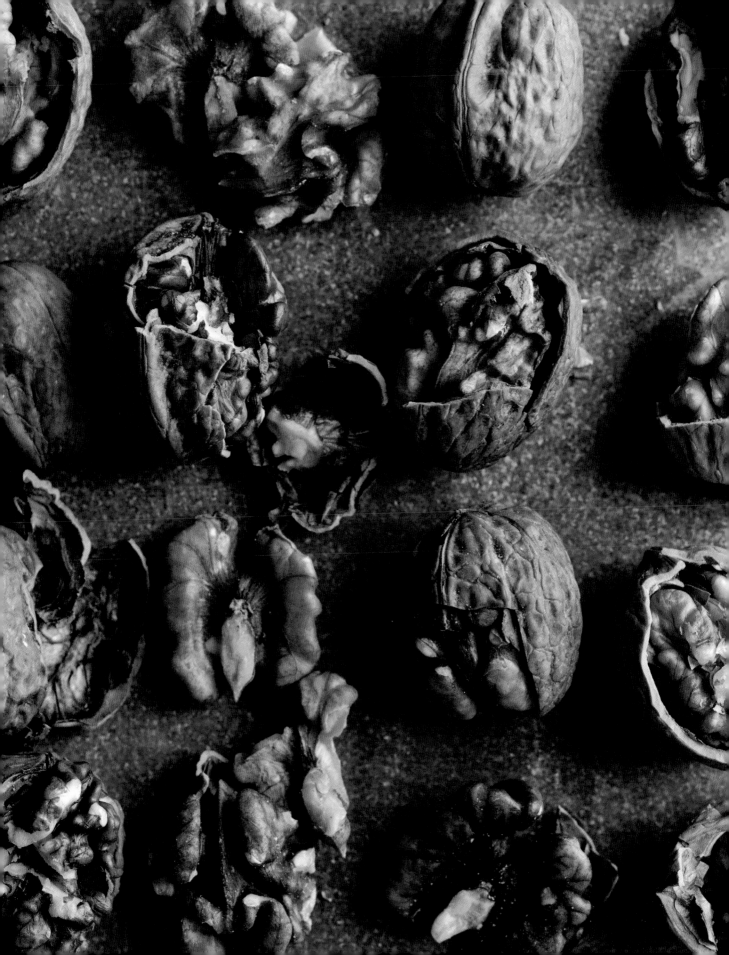

INDEX

F

Falafel Sliders, Beet, *122*, 123
Fasts, 221, 248
Fat flush, 217–23
    about, 217
    Dr. Bhatia and, xv
    Dr. Bhatia Q&A, 218–22
    Food Shortlist, 223
    goopified Menu, 223
    go-to snacks, 223
    sugar withdrawal, dealing with, 221
    See also Weight loss
Fats, dietary
    avoiding polyunsaturated oils, 249
    healthy choices, 220
Faux Meat Beet Tacos, 100, *101*
Fennel
    Italian Chicken Salad with Grilled
        Asparagus, 58
    Mediterranean Salmon en Papillote, *112*, 113
Fermented foods, 223, 234, 235, 240, 243
    fat flush go-to snacks with sauerkraut, 223
Fiber, 220, 254
Fish
    Fish *en Papillote*, 2 Ways, 111–15
    Fish Tacos on Jicama "Tortillas," *97*,
        98, 99
    See also specific types of fish
Fish oil, 234, 247
Fish sauce
    brand recommended, xvi
    Chicken Larb Lettuce Cups, 87
    Coconut Chicken Soup, 41
    Crunchy Summer Rolls, *90*, 91
Five-Spice Salmon Burgers, 125
Flaxseeds, 228
    Seed Cracker, 203, *203*
Food allergy, 234
Food cravings, 218
Food sensitivities, xi, xii, xv, 234
    elimination diet, xii
    testing for, xii
    See also Gluten
Foods excluded from recipes, xv
Food Shortlists
    adrenal support, 235
    Ayurveda cleanse, 255
    Candida reset, 243
    fat flush, 223
    heart health, 249
    heavy metal detox, 229

Fruits, 220, 223
    astringent, 252
    Ayurveda cleanse and, 252, 254, 255
    lectin-containing types, 246, 249
    nonorganic, 229
    See also specific fruits
Fungal infections, 238, 239
    See also Candida

G

Garam masala
    Chickpea & Kale Curry, 141
    Roasted Kabocha Soup, *34*, 35
    Sheet Pan Chicken Curry, *118*, 119
    Spinach & Pea Curry, 146
Garden Salad with Aquafaba Ranch Dressing, 59
Garlic, 242, 243
    Chicken & Cabbage Dim Sum, *142–44*, 145
    Chickpea & Escarole Soup, 51
    heavy metal detox and, 228
    Kale Aglio e Olio, *132*, 133
    Lemony Garlic Aquafaba Sauce, 179
    Tahini Dressing, 189
Gazpacho
    Beet Gazpacho, 36, *37*
    Cucumber & Avocado Gazpacho, 40, *40*
Ghee, 220, 254
Ghrelin, 218
Ginger, 242
    for Ayurveda cleanse go-to snack, 255
    Brown Rice, Turmeric & Spinach Porridge,
        48, *49*
    for Candida reset go-to snacks, 243
    Chicken & Cabbage Dim Sum, *142–44*, 145
    Chicken Meatball Pho, 42
    Clean Carrot Soup, *32*, 33
    Coconut Aminos Sauce, 186
    Coconut Chicken Soup, 41
    Five-Spice Salmon Burgers, 125
    Ginger & Cilantro Tea, 170
    Miso-Ginger Dressing, 188
    Roasted Kabocha Soup, *34*, 35
Glucagon, 233
Gluten, xi, xv, 95, 223, 235
    Ayurveda cleanse and, 255
    elimination diet and, 234
    sensitivity or allergy, xv
Glyphosate, 247
Goop.com
    Candida resources, 237
    recipes on, 140

Grains
    avoiding, 16, 240, 243, 247
    cauliflower rice as substitute, 69
    gluten-free, 254
    Grain Bowls, 3 Ways, 64–68
    lectins and, 247, 249
    mycotoxin residue and, 229
    See also specific grains
Grapefruit, 235
    for Ayurveda cleanse go-to snack, 255
Grapeseed extract, 248
Greek Salad, 62
Greens, 220, 223, 227, 229
    Easy Frittata, *20*, 21
    Eggs and Greens, 3 Ways, 18–23
    Poached Eggs over Sautéed Greens, 22, *23*
    Veggie Scramble, *2*, 19
Green tea, 221, 248
Grilled Chicken Salad with Miso Dressing, 55
Gundry, Steven
    about, 245
    Center for Restorative Medicine, 245
    Dr. Gundry's Diet Evolution, 245
    limiting lectins, 35, 245, 246
    The Plant Paradox, 245
    The Plant Paradox Cookbook, 245
    Q&A with, 246–48
    Vital Red supplement by, 248
Gut
    adrenal fatigue and, 233
    damage from anti-inflammatory drugs, 247
    damage from glyphosate, 247
    detox of, 220
    fasting and, 248
    health of, xii
    leaky gut, xii, 238, 239
    polyphenols and, 247
    rebalancing microbiome, xv
    resetting, 221
    serotonin and, 233

H

Halibut
    Fish Tacos on Jicama "Tortillas," *97*, *98*, 99
    Halibut en Papillote with Lemon,
        Mushrooms & Toasted Sesame Oil,
        114, *115*
Heart health, xii, 245–49
    Dr. Gundry Q&A, 246–48
    Dr. Gundry's program, 246
    exercise and, 248

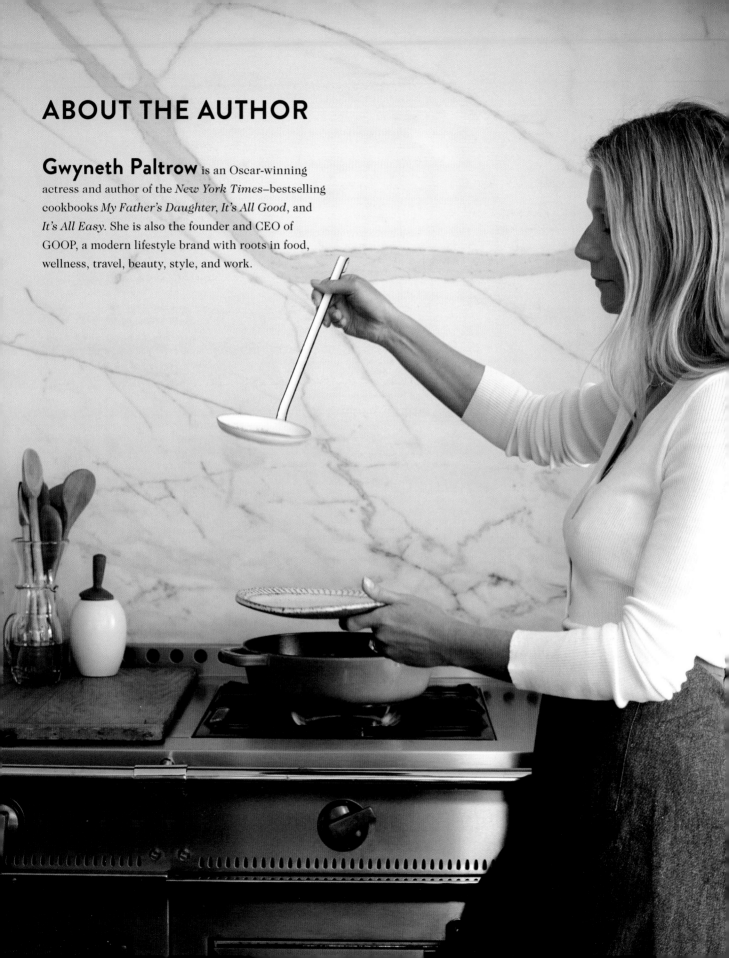

ABOUT THE AUTHOR

Gwyneth Paltrow is an Oscar-winning actress and author of the *New York Times*–bestselling cookbooks *My Father's Daughter*, *It's All Good*, and *It's All Easy*. She is also the founder and CEO of GOOP, a modern lifestyle brand with roots in food, wellness, travel, beauty, style, and work.

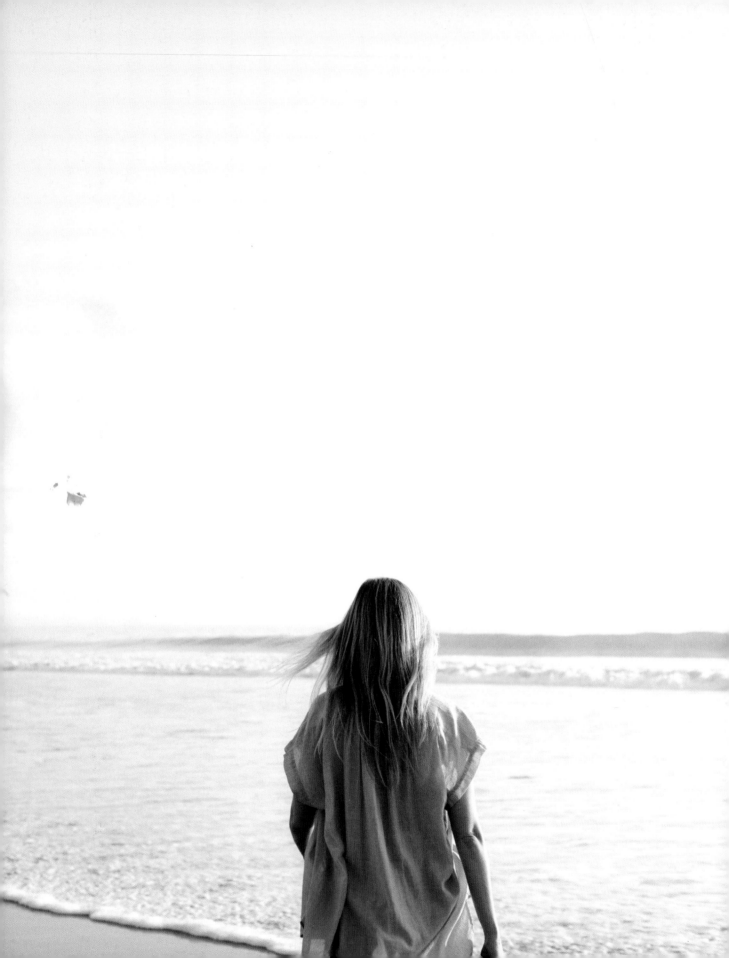